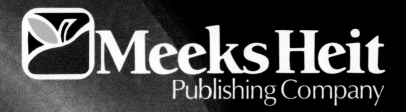

Meeks Heit
Publishing Company

Totally
Awesome®
Health

Linda Meeks
The Ohio State University

Philip Heit
The Ohio State University

Meeks Heit Publishing Company
Editorial, Sales, and Customer Service
6833 Clark State Road
Blacklick, OH 43004
(614) 939-1111

Director of Editorial: Julie DeVillers
Managing Editor: Ginger Panico
Project Editors: Heather L. Allen, Teri A. Curtis
Director of Illustration: Deborah Rubenstein
Director of Graphics: Elizabeth S. Kim
Graphics Associate: DanniElena Wolfe Hernández
Art Consultant: Jim Brower
Director of Production: Sally Meckling
Designer: Mary Geer
Photographers: Roman Sapecki, Lew Lause
Illustrators: Jennifer King, Dave Odell
Poetry Contributor: Katherine Shwed

Unit 10 outlines emergency care procedures that reflect the standard of knowledge and accepted practices in the United States at the time this book was published. It is the teacher's responsibility to stay informed of changes in emergency care procedures in order to teach current accepted practices. The teacher also can recommend that students gain complete, comprehensive training from courses offered by the American Red Cross.

Printed in the United States of America

3 4 5 6 7 8 9 10 99

Library of Congress Catalog Number: 98-066099

ISBN: 1-886693-58-7

About Meeks Heit Publishing Company

Professor Linda Meeks   **Dr. Philip Heit**

Linda Meeks and Philip Heit are emeritus professors of Health Education in the College of Education at The Ohio State University. Linda and Philip are America's most widely published health education co-authors. They have collaborated for more than 20 years, co-authoring more than 200 health books that are used by millions of students preschool through college. Together, they have helped state departments of education as well as thousands of school districts develop comprehensive school health education curricula. Their books and curricula are used throughout the United States as well as in Canada, Japan, Mexico, England, Puerto Rico, Spain, Egypt, Jordan, Saudi Arabia, Bermuda, and the Virgin Islands. Linda and Philip train professors as well as educators in state departments of education and school districts. Their book, *Comprehensive School Health Education: Totally Awesome® Strategies for Teaching Health,* is the most widely used book for teacher training in colleges, universities, and school districts. Thousands of teachers throughout the world have participated in their Totally Awesome® Teacher Training Workshops. Linda and Philip have been the keynote speakers for many teacher institutes and wellness conferences. They are personally and professionally committed to the health and well-being of youth.

Contributing Consultant

Susan Wooley, Ph.D., CHES
Executive Director
American School Health Association
Kent, Ohio

Advisory Board

Catherine M. Balsley, Ed.D., CHES
Curriculum Coordinator for
  Comprehensive Health Education
School District of Philadelphia
Philadelphia, Pennsylvania

Gary English, Ph.D., CHES
Associate Professor of Health Education
Department of Health Promotion and
  Human Movement
Ithaca College
Ithaca, New York

Deborah Fortune, Ph.D., CHES
Director of HIV/AIDS Project
Association for the Advancement of
  Health Education
Reston, Virginia

Alison Gardner, M.S., R.D.
Public Health Nutrition Chief
Vermont Department of Health
Burlington, Vermont

Sheryl Gotts, M.S.
Curriculum Specialist
Office of Health and Physical Education
Milwaukee Public Schools
Milwaukee, Wisconsin

David Lohrmann, Ph.D., CHES
Project Director
The Evaluation Consultation Center
Academy for Educational Development
Washington, D.C.

Judy Loper, Ph.D., R.D., L.D.
Director
Central Ohio Nutrition Center
Columbus, Ohio

Deborah Miller, Ph.D., CHES
Professor and Health Coordinator
College/University of Charleston
Charleston, South Carolina

Joanne Owens-Nauslar, Ed.D.
Director of Professional Development
American School Health Association
Kent, Ohio

Linda Peveler, M.S.
Health Teacher
Columbiana Middle School
Shelby County Public Schools
Birmingham, Alabama

LaNaya Ritson, M.S., CHES
Instructor, Department of Health Education
Western Oregon University
Monmouth, Oregon

John Rohwer, Ed.D.
Professor, Department of Health Education
Bethel College
St. Paul, Minnesota

Michael Schaffer, M.A.
Supervisor of Health
  Education K–12
Prince George's County
  Public Schools
Upper Marlboro, Maryland

Sherman Sowby, Ph.D., CHES
Professor, Health Science
California State University at Fresno
Fresno, California

Mae Waters, Ph.D., CHES
Executive Director Comprehensive School
  Health Programs Training Center
Florida State University
Tallahassee, Florida

Dee Wengert, Ph.D., CHES
Professor, Department of Health Science
Towson State University
Towson, Maryland

Medical Reviewers

Donna Bacchi, M.D., M.P.H.
Associate Professor of
  Pediatrics
Director, Division of
  Community Pediatrics
Texas Tech University
  Health Sciences Center
Lubbock, Texas

Albert J. Hart, Jr., M.D.
Mid-Ohio OB-GYN, Inc.
Westerville, Ohio

Reviewers

Kymm Ballard, M.A.
Physical Education, Athletics,
  and Sports Medicine
  Consultant
North Carolina Department
  of Public Instruction
Raleigh, North Carolina

Kay Bridges
Health Educator
Gaston County Public Schools
Gastonia, North Carolina

Reba Bullock, M.Ed.
Health Education Curriculum
  Specialist
Baltimore City Public Schools
Baltimore, Maryland

Anthony S. Catalano, Ph.D.
K–12 Health Coordinator
Melrose Public Schools
Melrose, Massachusetts

Galen Cole, M.P.H., Ph.D.
Division of Health
  Communication
Office of the Director
Centers for Disease Control
  and Prevention
Atlanta, Georgia

Brian Colwell, Ph.D.
Professor
Department of HLKN
Texas A&M University
College Station, Texas

Tommy Fleming, Ph.D.
Director of Health and
  Physical Education
Texas Education Agency
Austin, Texas

Denyce Ford, M.Ed., Ph.D.
Coordinator, Comprehensive
  School Health Education
District of Columbia Public
  Schools
Washington, D.C.

Elizabeth Gallun, M.A.
Supervisor of Drug Programs
Prince George's County
  Public Schools
Upper Marlboro, Maryland

Linda Harrill-Rudisill, M.A.
Chairperson of Health
  Education
Southwest Middle Schools
Gastonia, North Carolina

Janet Henke
Middle School Team Leader
Baltimore County Public
  Schools
Baltimore, Maryland

Russell Henke
Coordinator of Health
Montgomery County Public
  Schools
Rockville, Maryland

Larry Herrold, M.S.
Supervisor, Office of Health
  and Physical Education
  K–12
Baltimore County Schools
Baltimore, Maryland

Susan Jackson, B.S., M.A.
Health Promotion Specialist
Healthworks, Wake Medical
  Center
Raleigh, North Carolina

Joe Leake, CHES
Curriculum Specialist
Baltimore City Public Schools
Baltimore, Maryland

Debra Ogden, M.A.
Coordinator of Health,
  Physical Education, Driver
  Education, and Safe and
  Drug-Free Programs
Collier County Public
  Schools
Naples, Florida

Diane S. Scalise, R.N., M.S.
Coordinator, Health
  Education Services
The School Board of
  Broward County
Fort Lauderdale, Florida

Merita Thompson, Ed.D.
Professor of Health
  Education
Eastern Kentucky University
Richmond, Kentucky

Linda Wright, M.A.
Project Director
HIV/AIDS Education
  Program
District of Columbia
  Public Schools
Washington, D.C.

Unit 1

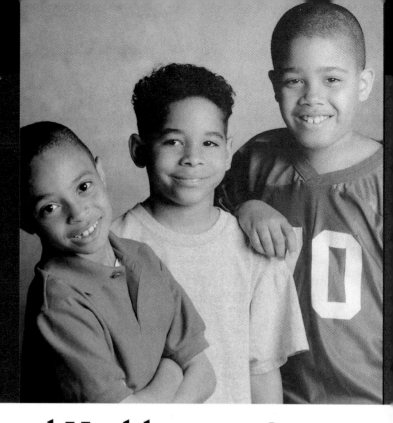

Mental and Emotional Health

Unit 2

Family and Social Health

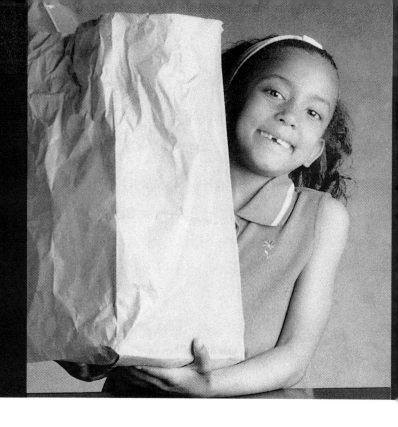

Unit 3

Growth and Development

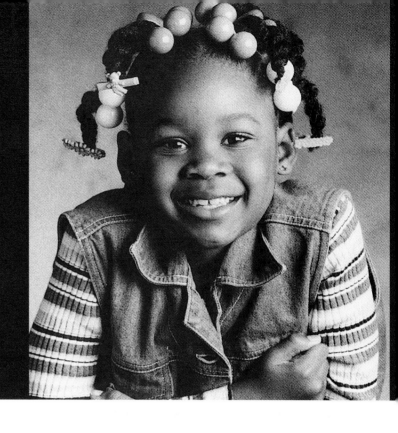

Unit 4

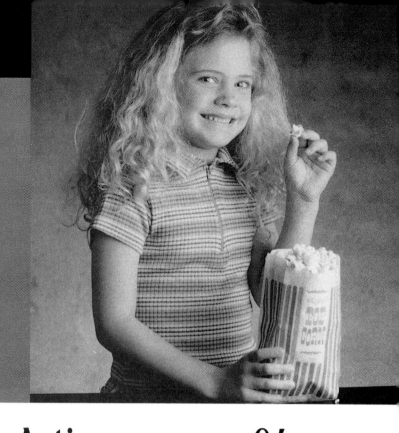

Nutrition

Unit 5

Personal Health and Physical Activity

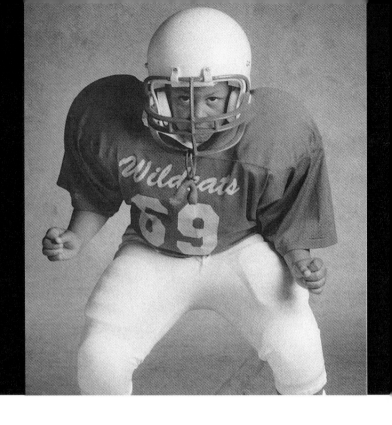

Unit 6

Alcohol, Tobacco, and Other Drugs

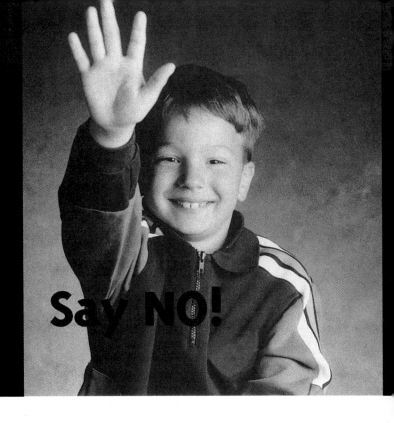

Say NO!

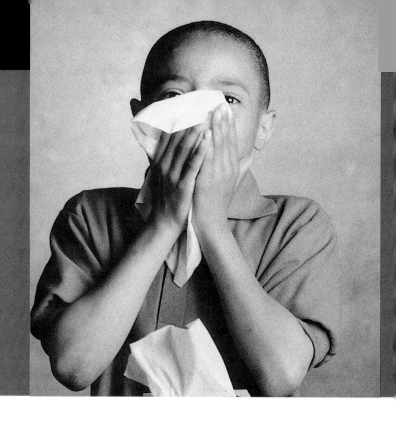

Unit 7

Communicable and Chronic Diseases

Unit 8

Consumer and Community Health

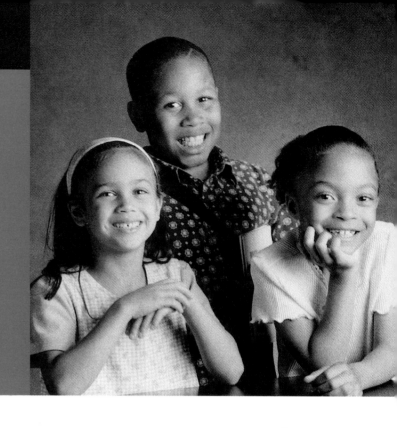

Unit 9

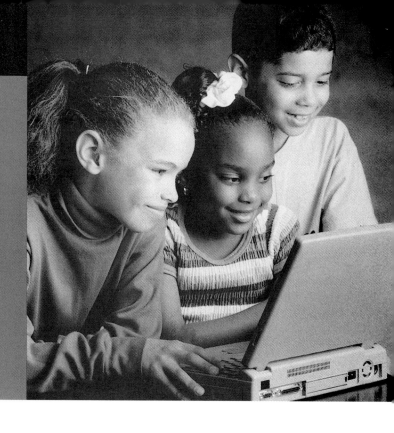

Environmental Health

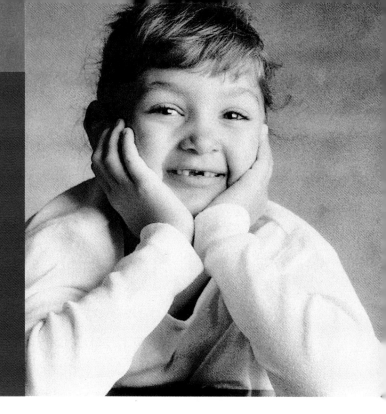

Unit 10

Injury Prevention and Safety

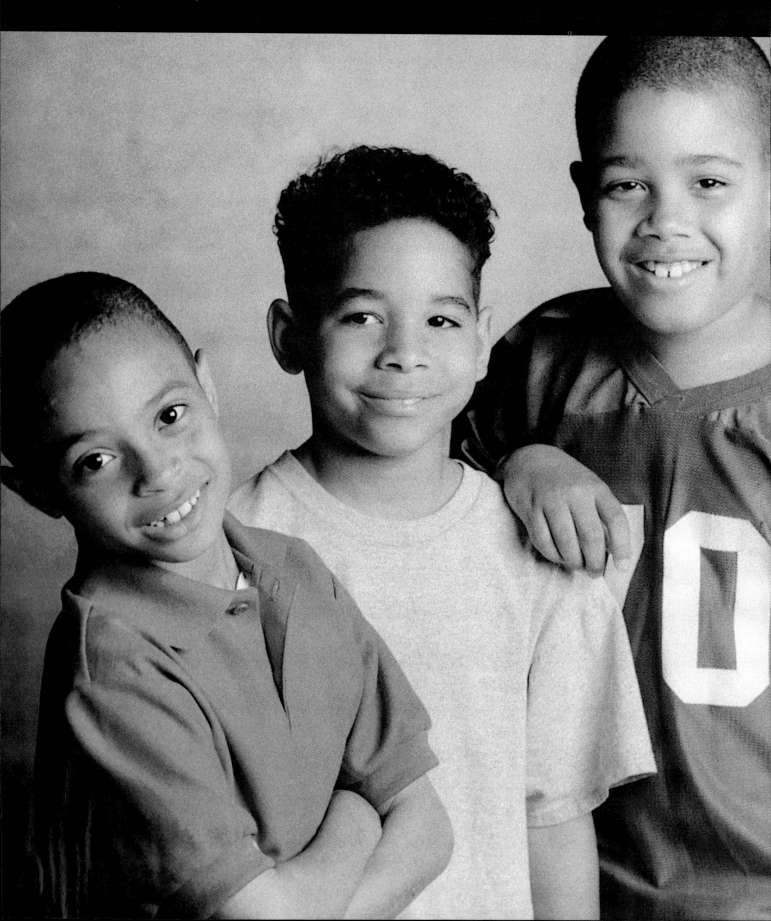

Mental and Emotional Health

Say YES to Good Health

Vocabulary

health: the condition of your body, mind, and relationships.

life skill: a healthful action you learn and practice for life.

responsible: to be in charge of doing something.

health behavior contract: a written plan to help you practice a life skill.

Life Skills

- I will take responsibility for my health.
- I will practice life skills for health.

Suppose a friend asks you to go to a movie. You say YES to your friend. Then another friend asks you to bike. You have already promised to go to the movie. You must say NO when the friend asks you to bike. When you say YES, you make a promise to do something. This means you must say NO to anything that would cause you to break your promise.

The Lesson Objectives

- Tell reasons to say YES to good health.
- Name the three parts of total health.
- Make a health behavior contract for a life skill.

Why Say YES to Good Health?

Health is the condition of your body, mind, and relationships. A **life skill** is a healthful action you learn and practice for life. Here is how you say YES to health. You make a promise to practice life skills. You keep your promise for the rest of your life.

This book has many lessons in it. Each lesson gives you facts. Each lesson tells you how to practice one or more life skills. Here are some of the life skills in this book.

- I will get plenty of physical activity.
- I will have regular checkups.
- I will get enough rest and sleep.
- I will eat healthful meals and snacks.
- I will work to have healthful friendships.
- I will work to have healthful family relationships.
- I will not drink alcohol.
- I will not use tobacco.

There are reasons to say YES to good health. You can play sports and games without getting tired. You know how to make and keep friends. You do not get sick as often. You enjoy activities with friends. You stay in a good mood most of the time.

YES to Health Means NO to Wrong Actions

Suppose someone asks you to take a puff of a cigarette. But you have said YES to health. You have promised to practice life skills now and for the rest of your life. You must say NO. You must not take a puff of the cigarette. Saying YES to health is a very important promise. You will be glad you made this promise.

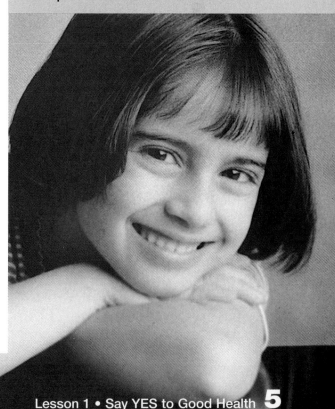

What Are the Three Parts of Total Health?

Have you ever put a puzzle together? If you have, you put the pieces together first. Then you could see the whole picture. What if you did not have one of the puzzle pieces? Then you would not be able to see the whole picture.

There are three parts of total health. The three parts must fit together for you to have total health. Suppose one part of health is missing. Then you do not have total health.

Physical Health

Physical health is how well your body works. You can say YES to having physical health. Eat breakfast and choose healthful snacks. Get plenty of physical activity. Get enough rest and sleep. Then you will not tire easily. You will have a healthy heart.

Mental and Emotional Health

Mental and emotional health is how well your mind works and how you show your feelings. You can say YES to having this kind of health. Work crossword puzzles. Check out library books and read them. Then your mind will work well. Share your feelings with your parents or guardian. Write about your feelings when you are upset. Then you show feelings in healthful ways.

Total Health Has Three Parts

The three parts are like pieces of a puzzle. They fit together to make a picture of health. The three parts of total health are:

- Physical health
- Mental and emotional health
- Social health

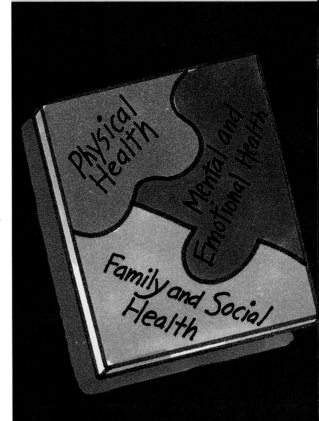

Family and Social Health

Family and social health is how well you get along with your family and others. You can say YES to having family and social health. Spend time with family members. Use table manners when you eat dinner. Help your family with chores. Follow family rules. Then you will get along well with your family. Listen to your friends when they speak. Be fair when you play games on the playground. Then you will get along well with others.

You Are Responsible for Total Health

To be **responsible** (ri·SPAHN·suh·buhl) is to be in charge of doing something. Your parents or guardian are responsible for you. They help you practice life skills. For example, they help you pick foods for breakfast. They tell you when to go to bed so you get enough sleep. You must cooperate with your parents or guardian. You must be responsible for total health.

Your Total Health Puzzle

Life Skill

- I will take responsibility for my health.

Materials: Construction paper, markers or crayons, scissors

Directions: Draw a puzzle outline on construction paper. The puzzle should have three pieces. Cut out the three pieces. Write "physical health" on one piece. Write "mental and emotional health" on one piece. Write "family and social health" on one piece. Make drawings on each piece. For example, you might draw a book for "mental and emotional health." Give your puzzle to a classmate to put together.

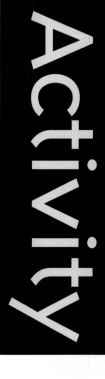

Activity

How Do I Make a Health Behavior Contract?

A **health behavior contract** is a written plan to help you practice a life skill.

Copy the health behavior contract on a separate sheet of paper.

DO NOT WRITE IN THIS BOOK.

Health Behavior Contract

There are four steps to help you make a health behavior contract.

Name: _____ **Date:** _____

Life Skill: I will be well-groomed.

Effect on My Health: Grooming is having a neat and clean appearance. Good grooming helps keep my skin, hair, and nails clean. It keeps my hands clean. Then there will not be germs on them. I will be less likely to get sick.

My Plan: I will wash my hands often. Each time I wash my hands I will draw a smiley face on one of the fingers below.

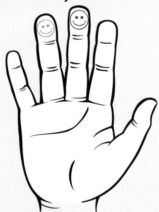

How My Plan Worked: Did I wash my hands often? Did I wash my hands after I used the restroom? Did I wash my hands before I ate food?

1. Tell the life skill you want to practice.

2. Tell how the life skill will affect your health.

3. Describe a plan you will follow and how you will keep track of your progress.

4. Tell how your plan worked.

High-Five

Life Skill

• I will practice life skills for health.

Materials: None

Directions: Look at the life skills on page 5. Look through your book to find other life skills. They are on the first page of each lesson.

1. **Pick a life skill you will promise to practice.** For example, you might choose the following one: "I will get plenty of physical activity."

2. **One classmate will stand and say the life skill he or she picked. This classmate will turn and give a second classmate a high-five. They will say "YES!"** For example, the classmate might say, "I will get plenty of physical activity."

3. **The second classmate will say a life skill and turn and give a high-five to a third classmate. They will say "YES!"** The second classmate might say this life skill: "I will get enough rest and sleep." Repeat and include other classmates.

Activity

Lesson 1

Review

Vocabulary

Write a separate sentence using each vocabulary word listed on page 4.

Health Content

1. What are reasons to say YES to good health? **page 5**

2. What are some life skills that are in your health book? **page 5**

3. What are the three parts of total health? **pages 6–7**

4. Who is responsible for your health? **page 7**

5. What are the four parts of a health behavior contract? **page 8**

Lesson 1 • Say YES to Good Health **9**

Pledge to Make Responsible Decisions

Vocabulary

responsible decision: a choice you will be proud of.

rule: a guide to help you do the right thing.

good character: telling the truth, showing respect, and being fair.

resistance skills: ways to say NO to wrong decisions.

peer: someone who is your age.

Life Skills

- I will make responsible decisions.
- I will use resistance skills when necessary.

A *decision* (di·SI·zhuhn) is a choice. Every day you make decisions that affect health. Suppose you decide to bike. Your choice helps your physical health. Suppose you decide to read a book. Your choice helps mental and emotional health. Suppose you decide to help your family wash dishes. Your choice helps family and social health. You can pledge to make responsible decisions.

The Lesson Objectives

- List six questions to ask before you make a decision.
- Explain how to use resistance skills.
- Explain what to do if a friend plans to do something wrong.

Making Responsible Decisions Sing-Along™

Life Skill

- I will **make responsible decisions.**

Materials: Guitar or piano (optional)

Directions: A **responsible decision** is a choice you will be proud of. The next two pages of this lesson tell you how to make a responsible decision. There are six questions to answer to help you. This song will help you remember the six questions.

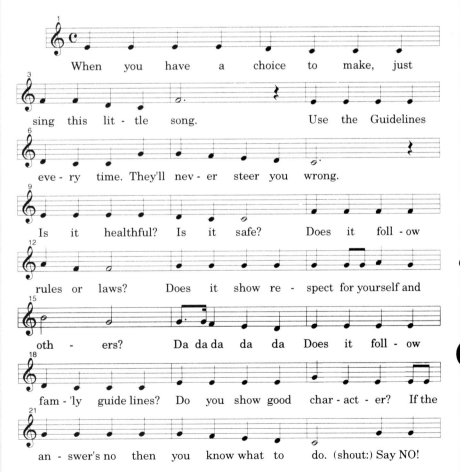

When you have a choice to make, just sing this lit-tle song. Use the Guidelines eve-ry time. They'll nev-er steer you wrong. Is it healthful? Is it safe? Does it foll-ow rules or laws? Does it show re-spect for yourself and oth-ers? Da da da da da Does it foll-ow fam-'ly guide lines? Do you show good char-act-er? If the an-swer's no then you know what to do. (shout:) Say NO!

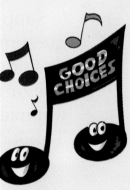

Activity

What Are Six Questions to Ask Before I Make a Decision?

Suppose you have a decision to make. Take time to think. Ask yourself questions. The *Guidelines for Making Responsible Decisions*™ are six questions to ask to help you make a responsible decision. Always ask these six questions. Just fill in the blanks.

The Guidelines for Making Responsible Decisions™

1. Is it healthful to _____?

2. Is it safe to _____?

3. Do I follow rules and laws if I _____?

4. Do I show respect for myself and others if I _____?

5. Do I follow my family's guidelines if I _____?

6. Do I show good character if I _____?

Suppose you answer YES to all six questions. Then you make a responsible decision. Suppose you answer NO to one or more of the six questions. You will make a wrong decision. STOP! Think of another choice.

Say YES to Rules!

A **rule** is a guide to help you do the right thing. Your family has rules. Your school has rules. When you follow rules, you do the right thing. When you break rules, bad things can happen. You might hurt yourself. You might hurt someone else. You might upset your parents or guardian.

Say YES to Good Character

Good character (KEHR·ik·tuhr) is telling the truth, showing respect, and being fair. Before you decide, stop and think. Do you plan to tell the truth? Do you plan to show respect? Do you plan to be fair?

Use... Guidelines for Making Responsible Decisions™

Situation:

You are playing kickball on the playground. The ball goes into the street. Your teammates want you to get the ball. They want you to run into the street.

Response:

Answer "yes" or "no" to each of the following questions. Explain each answer.

1. Is it healthful to run into the street?
2. Is it safe to run into the street?
3. Do you follow rules and laws if you run into the street?
4. Do you show respect for yourself and others if you run into the street?
5. Do you follow your family's guidelines if you run into the street?
6. Do you show good character if you run into the street?

What is the responsible decision to make?

These Questions Help You Make Hard Decisions

Suppose you have a hard decision to make. You are at home with your parents or guardian. You can talk over the decision with one of them. But suppose an adult is not with you. The *Guidelines for Making Responsible Decisions*™ help you know what is right. If you use them, no one will talk you into doing something wrong.

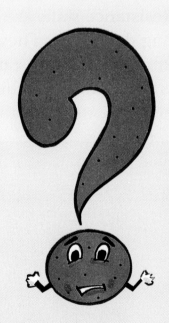

How Can I Use Resistance Skills?

Suppose a friend asks you to ice skate. The pond you will skate on is safe. There is an adult who watches while children skate on the pond. Your parents or guardian allow you to ice skate. What should you do? STOP and think ahead. Use the *Guidelines for Making Responsible Decisions*™. Answer the six questions. In this case, your answers will be YES. It is a responsible decision to ice skate.

Suppose a friend wants you to carve your name on your school desk. STOP and think ahead. Use the *Guidelines for Making Responsible Decisions*™. Answer the six questions. Then decide what to do. In this case, some of your answers will be NO. It is not a responsible decision to carve your name in your school desk.

Resistance skills are ways to say NO to wrong decisions. They are listed on the next page. Use resistance skills if a peer asks you to do something wrong. A **peer** is someone who is your age.

Help Your Friends Make Responsible Decisions

Suppose your friend plans to do something wrong. Do not go along with your friend's wrong actions. Tell your friend his or her actions will be wrong. Help your friend learn why. Mention the six questions. Ask your friend to answer them. Your friend will think well of you. Your friend will know you really care.

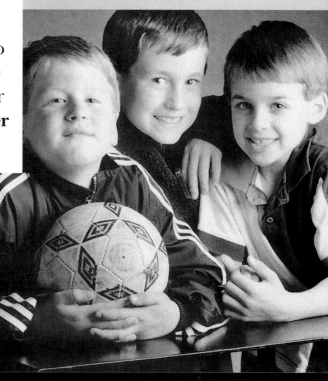

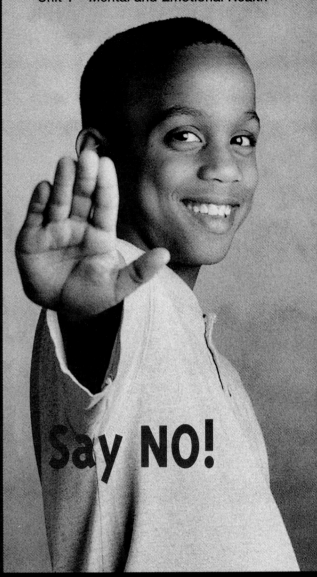

Resistance Skills

1. Say NO in a firm voice.

2. Give reasons for saying NO.

3. Match your actions with your words.

4. Keep away from situations in which peers might try to talk you into wrong decisions.

5. Keep away from peers who make wrong decisions.

6. Tell an adult if someone tries to talk you into a wrong decision.

7. Help your friends make responsible decisions.

Lesson 2

Review

Vocabulary

Write a separate sentence using each vocabulary word listed on page 10.

Health Content

1. What are six questions to ask before you make a decision? **page 12**

2. Why do you need to follow rules? **page 12**

3. What is good character? **page 12**

4. What should you do if a friend plans to do something wrong? **page 14**

5. What are seven resistance skills? **page 15**

Hang On to Good Character

Vocabulary

respect: thinking highly of someone.

willpower: the strength you need to do the right thing.

pay back: to make good for loss or damage.

pay forward: to pay back for wrongdoing by doing something kind for someone else.

hero: a person you look up to because of something the person has done or does.

Life Skill

● **I will show good character.**

Suppose a friend tells someone about you. Your friend describes what you are like. What do you think your friend would say? Would your friend say you have good character? This lesson is about good character. Do you know what good character is?

The Lesson Objectives

● Tell three actions that make up good character.

● Tell situations when you will need good character.

● Explain what to do if you do something wrong.

● Explain why your heroes should have good character.

What Are Three Actions That Make Up Good Character?

Good character is:

- telling the truth,
- showing respect,
- and being fair.

Pay attention to the three actions that make up good character. Choose these actions at all times.

Always tell the truth. Then people know they can count on you. Suppose you are tempted to stretch the truth. Do not think it is no big deal. Do not think it will be OK if you do not get caught. Any lie is wrong, even a small one. Suppose people find out that you lie. Then they will not trust you.

Always show respect for other people. **Respect** is thinking highly of someone. Treat other people the same way you want to be treated. Do not put down people who are different from you. Do not treat someone you do not like in wrong ways. If you show respect for other people, they are more likely to show respect for you.

Always be fair. Never cheat at games or on school work. Remember to take your turn. Never take anything that does not belong to you. Play by the rules.

Remind Yourself to Hang On to Good Character

Create a "Hang On to Good Character" hangtag.

A hangtag is a tag made of cardboard that is hung on a doorknob or other knob. Cut a hangtag out of cardboard. Use a marker. Write "Hang On to Good Character" at the top. Then write:

- I will tell the truth.
- I will show respect.
- I will be fair.

Put the hangtag on a doorknob or other knob. It can help remind you to hang on to good character.

What Are Situations When I Need Good Character?

Good character is something you need all the time. At times, it is easy to show good character. Sometimes it takes willpower. **Willpower** is the strength you need to do the right thing. Use willpower when you need to do so. Show good character in the following situations.

To make responsible decisions

Sometimes decisions are hard to make. You might be tempted to make a wrong decision. Good character helps you make a responsible decision.

To keep from giving in to a tempting situation
Sometimes you are tempted to do something wrong. Perhaps you know that no one will find out. Good character helps you overcome a tempting situation.

To admit something wrong you have done
Everybody makes mistakes. It is part of growing up. But it is not OK to cover up something wrong you have done. Good character helps you admit you did something wrong. It helps you make up for what you did.

To prevent violence if someone wants you to fight
You will be in situations where other people want to pick a fight. It might be during a game. It might be on the school playground. Good character keeps you from fighting.

Friends Who Have Good Character

Always choose friends who have good character. You can count on these friends. They:

- make responsible decisions.
- do not give in to tempting situations.
- admit something wrong they have done.
- protect against violence by not fighting.

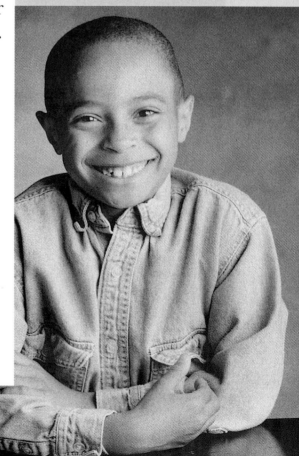

What Should I Do If I Do Something Wrong?

Suppose you do something wrong. You might have done something you knew was wrong at the time. You might have done something wrong by accident. When you do something wrong, you must correct your actions.

Pay back Suppose your friend just got a new game. You borrow it and lose one of the pieces. To **pay back** is to make good for loss or damage. One kind of payback involves replacing something. You might give your friend money to replace the missing piece. You might give your friend money to buy a new game.

Another kind of payback involves paying someone back with time or work. Suppose you ride your bike and run over your neighbor's flowers by accident. You might offer to spend a few hours weeding the garden.

Pay forward Suppose you cannot pay back someone you harmed. To **pay forward** is to pay back for wrongdoing by doing something kind for someone else. Maybe there was a girl at your school who you teased last year. You feel badly, but she has moved. This year there is a new boy at school. Some classmates tease him. You ask them to stop.

Saying You Are Sorry

Suppose you cause someone harm. It is not enough to pay back with money or other actions. Say you are sorry and mean it. The other person will be more satisfied if you explain you are sorry.

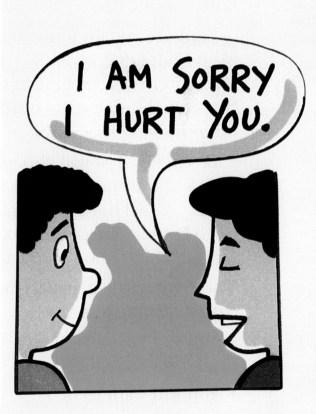

Why Should My Heroes Have Good Character?

A **hero** is a person you look up to because of something the person has done or does. Suppose you love baseball. You might watch baseball on TV. Your parents or guardian might take you to a professional baseball game. The pitcher of your favorite team might be a hero. You look up to the pitcher because he wins so many games.

Suppose you like science. One of your heroes might be a famous scientist. Perhaps this scientist wrote many books. You look up to this scientist because she knows so much.

Suppose you go to movies. There is a movie star you like a lot. This movie star is a hero in several movies you see. He becomes a favorite of yours. You look up to him because of his acting.

Be careful how you choose your heroes. Think about the examples that were given. A real hero is a person you look up to because the person does something well AND has good character, too.

Your heroes should have good character.

• You will know examples of good character.

• You will want to be known for having good character.

Everyday Heroes

Think about the real heroes in your life. These are the people who do things well and have good character. Your parents or guardian might be real heroes. They might work very hard at being parents. They might show good character. Your teacher, principal, and school nurse might be real heroes, too.

Be careful when you choose a hero. Look up to adults who are good at something AND have good character. Then you will want to have good character, too.

Character Awards

Life Skill

● I will show good character.

Materials: Paper, pencil, markers; computer and computer paper (optional)

Directions: The following activity gives you a chance to praise a person for good character.

1. **Put up someone you know for a character award.** You might have seen awards shows on TV. Awards are given for outstanding performances. Actors and actresses win awards. People who write music might win an award. Think of a person you know who has good character. You will put this person up for a character award.

2. **Write a speech to tell why you chose this person.** Tell at least three reasons why you put the person up for a character award. Your speech should talk your classmates into voting for the person you chose.

3. **Present your speech to the class.**

4. **Give a copy of your speech to the person you put up.**

Activity

Lesson 3

Review

Vocabulary

Write a separate sentence using each vocabulary word listed on page 16.

Health Content

1. What are three actions that make up good character? **page 17**

2. What are situations in which you need good character? **page 18**

3. How can you pay back if you do something wrong? **page 19**

4. How can you pay forward if you do something wrong? **page 19**

5. Why should your heroes have good character? **page 20**

Stay in a Good Mood

Vocabulary

mood: the way you feel at a certain time.

self-concept: the feeling you have about yourself.

addiction: letting a drug or habit control you.

feelings: the ways you feel inside.

I-message: a healthful way to say or write about feelings.

Life Skills

- I will choose behaviors to have a healthy mind.
- I will communicate in healthful ways.

Your **mood** is the way you feel at a certain time. Many things can cause changes in your mood. Your health can change your mood. Physical activity can change your mood. The ways you express feelings can change your mood.

The Lesson Objectives

- Discuss ways to stay in a good mood.
- Discuss ways to keep your mind healthy.
- Tell three questions to ask to help understand your feelings.
- Write an I-message to say angry feelings.
- Tell how to work things out if you are angry with someone.

What Are Ways to Stay in a Good Mood?

Most likely you have been around someone who was in a bad mood. The person might have been grumpy. The person might have been "down in the dumps." You probably have been in a bad mood. Did you know there are ways to stay in a good mood?

Get plenty of physical activity. Physical activity can make your mood better. *Beta-endorphins* (BAY·tuh·en·DOR·fuhns) are substances that make you feel good. Physical activity causes your body to make them. They get into your blood. They change your mood.

Work to do something well. Your **self-concept** is the feeling you have about yourself. When you do something well, you feel proud. You are satisfied with yourself. This helps you stay in a good mood.

Spend time with people who care about you. People who care about you help you feel important. They cheer you up if you are down in the dumps. They remind you that things will get better.

Do something for someone who is having hard times. It helps you see the things that are going well for you. You see that some of the things that bother you are not so bad after all.

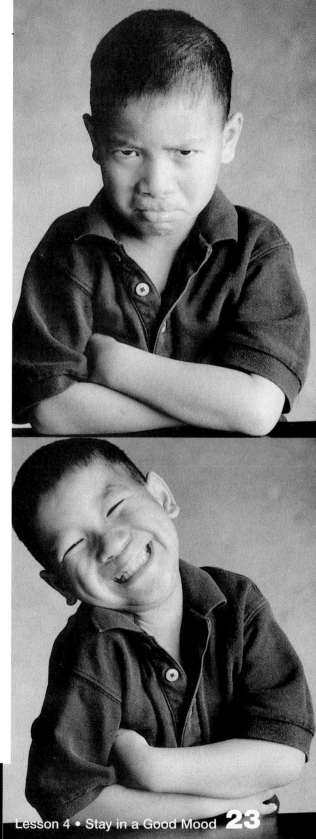

What Are Ways to Keep My Mind Healthy?

You must keep your mind in top condition. Pay attention to these ways to keep your mind healthy.

Get plenty of physical activity.

Physical activity keeps fat off the walls of your arteries. Then blood flows more smoothly through them. Blood flows to the arteries in your brain. Your brain cells get oxygen to do their work.

Get plenty of rest and sleep.

Your body would get too tired without rest and sleep. Your mind cannot keep working without rest and sleep. You think clearly when you have had rest and sleep.

Stay away from harmful drugs.

Alcohol slows down the activity of brain cells. You will not think clearly if you drink alcohol. Marijuana changes how you think. You will not think clearly if you use marijuana.

Get fresh air if you use cleaning products, paint, or glue.

Fumes from these products can harm brain cells. They can change how you think and feel.

Stay away from addictions.

An **addiction** (uh·DIK·shuhn) is letting a drug or habit control you. Children who have an addiction feel they have to do a certain thing. They allow something to control their mind. An addiction is a sickness. *Television addiction* is being unable to stop watching TV when you should be doing something else. Your mind is controlled by the TV. You are glued in front of the TV and forget to do other things. This is not healthful.

Work to Have a Good Memory

Your memory is your ability to remember things. Work to have a good memory. Play games like Concentration. Concentration is a card game in which you shuffle cards and put them face down. Then you turn two cards over to try to get a match. You keep the two cards if they match. You put them back face down if you do not. You try very hard to remember where you put the cards face down. Then you can get a match on your next try. You take turns with a partner. The person who has the most matches wins.

What Questions Can I Ask to Help Understand My Feelings?

To have a healthy mind, you need to show feelings in healthful ways. Everyone has feelings. **Feelings** are the ways you feel inside. You have feelings about everything that happens to you. You can show your feelings in healthful ways.

You might be sad when a friend moves away. Writing a note to your friend can help show your feelings in a healthful way. You might be happy when your team wins a soccer game. You might smile and jump for joy to show your happiness.

Questions you can ask to help you understand your feelings are:

• **What am I feeling?**

• **Why do I feel this way?**

• **How might I show this feeling in a healthful way?**

Suppose a classmate pushes you while you are standing in line. What are you feeling? You are feeling angry. Why do you feel this way? You feel angry because your classmate pushed you. How might you show this feeling in a healthful way? Pushing back could cause a fight. You decide to tell your classmate you are angry because he pushed you. You can ask your classmate to say he is sorry.

Kinds of Feelings
happy
sad
disappointed
angry
joyful
depressed

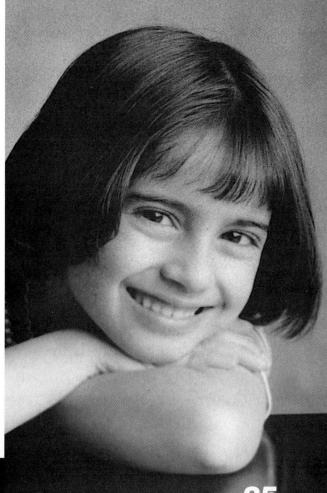

How Can I Say or Write About Angry Feelings?

Suppose you are angry. You have angry feelings when you are really upset with someone. You can say or write about your angry feelings. The other person can respond to your angry feelings.

An **I-message** is a healthful way to say or write about feelings. You can use I-messages to say or write about angry feelings. You just need practice. There are three things to put in an I-message. They are:

- what happened or is happening,
- how it affects you,
- how you feel about it.

Suppose a friend cuts in line in front of you. You want your friend to know how angry you are. You can put together an I-message.

- **What happened:** You cut in line.
- **How it affects you:** It is not fair.
- **How you feel about it:** I am angry.

Now put the I-message into a sentence you could say to your friend.

"When you cut in line, it is not fair and I am angry."

In this situation, you say the I-message to your friend. Sometimes you write I-messages. You might write a note to someone after something happens that makes you angry.

How to Work Things Out If You Are Angry with Someone

Step 1: Share your feelings.

Step 2: Tell what you want to happen to make things better.

Suppose you share the I-message on this page with your friend who cut in line. Your friend knows how you feel. You also might tell what you want to happen to make things better. You might say, "I would like you to go to the end of the line."

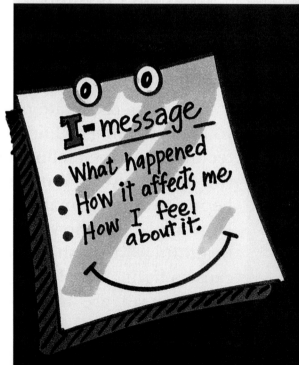

I-message
- What happened
- How it affects me
- How I feel about it.

Collage of Feelings

Life Skill

● I will communicate in healthful ways.

Materials: Poster board, magazines with pictures of faces, glue, scissors

Directions: Complete the following activity to see different feelings people have.

1. **Cut out magazine pictures of faces to show different feelings.** Try to find faces that show lots of different feelings. You might find faces that show being happy, being sad, and being angry.

2. **Make a collage from the faces that you cut out.** A collage is made by gluing together all the faces on the poster board. You can put them together in any design you want.

3. **Show your collage to the class and name the feelings that are shown on the faces.**

Activity

Lesson 4

Review

Vocabulary

Write a separate sentence using each vocabulary word listed on page 22.

Health Content

1. What are ways you can stay in a good mood? **page 23**

2. What are ways to keep your mind healthy? **page 24**

3. What are three questions you can ask to help understand your feelings? **page 25**

4. How can you say or write about angry feelings? **page 26**

5. How can you work things out if you are angry with someone? **page 26**

Soaking Up Stress

Vocabulary

stress: the response to any demand on your mind and body.

stressor: anything that causes stress.

healthful stress: stress that helps you perform well and stay healthy.

harmful stress: stress that harms health or causes you to perform poorly.

beta-endorphins: substances that make you feel good.

Life Skills

- I will have a plan for stress.
- I will bounce back from hard times.

Stress is the response to any demand on your mind and body. Everyone feels stress. There might be stress in your life each day. What causes stress? How does stress affect you? Do you know how to control stress?

The Lesson Objectives

- Name kinds of stressors.
- Name body changes caused by stress.
- Explain healthful stress.
- Explain harmful stress.
- Discuss ways to control stress.

What Are Kinds of Stressors?

A **stressor** (STRE·suhr) is anything that causes stress. Stressors can affect you more or less than they affect someone else. There are many kinds of stressors.

Having to perform can be a stressor. Suppose you have to sing in front of your classmates. You might worry that you will not sing well.

Something in the environment can be a stressor. Your *environment* (in·VY·ruhn·muhnt) is everything that is around you. Suppose the room you are in is very noisy. The noise bothers you when you try to read. You have to read a paragraph more than once to understand it. Noise is a stressor.

Suppose the temperature is very cold. You must wear a scarf over your nose to keep from breathing air that is too cold. Your fingers and toes are very cold. Very cold and very hot temperatures can be stressors.

Being sick can be a stressor. Suppose you have the flu. You have a fever and headache. Your body works hard to try to get well. This is a stressor.

Having a disagreement with a friend can be a stressor. Suppose you disagree with a friend and do not work it out. You worry about your friendship. You do not sleep. This is a stressor.

Body Changes When You Have Stress

Suppose you have stress. Stress causes body changes. These body changes get you ready for quick action.

- Your heart beats faster to pump blood to your muscles.
- You breathe faster to get more oxygen.
- Sugar stored in your body goes into the blood for energy.
- Your mouth might get dry.
- Your hands might get sweaty.
- Your muscles might feel tight.

What Is Healthful Stress?

Healthful stress is stress that helps you perform well and stay healthy. Let's look at an example of healthful stress. Suppose you are the pitcher on a baseball team. The bases are loaded. The next batter is ready. You must strike this batter out to win the game.

You feel stress. You breathe faster to get more oxygen. Your heart beats faster to get blood with oxygen to your muscles. Sugar is released into your blood. The sugar gives you extra energy. These body changes help you perform well. You throw two strikes. Then you throw a ball. But you do not lose your focus. Stress helps you pull yourself together to throw your best pitch. You strike the batter out.

The body changes you had from stress helped you perform well. They did not cause you to get too tired. After the game, you were not under stress. The body changes from stress are gone. Your heart rate is back to normal. Your breathing is back to normal. There is not extra sugar in your blood.

Healthful Stress Can:

- help you perform well.
- give you energy.

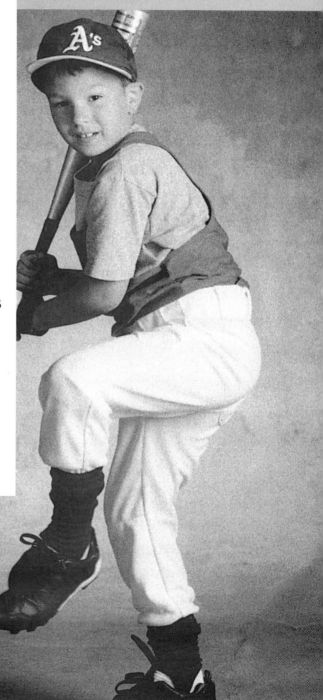

What Is Harmful Stress?

Harmful stress is stress that harms health or causes you to perform poorly. If harmful stress lasts, you can get diseases. Let's look at examples of harmful stress.

Suppose you are going to be in a school play. You have not practiced the lines you will say. You worry that you will not say your lines correctly. You do not sleep the night before the play. The day of the play you are very tired. Your stomach is upset. You cannot remember your lines. Harmful stress caused you to perform poorly in the play.

Harmful stress also can cause disease. Let's look at what happens when harmful stress lasts a long time. Suppose a child's parent is very ill and does not get better. The child worries about her parent.

She does not sleep well for several weeks. She makes many mistakes in her schoolwork. Her grades go down. She gets headaches and stomachaches. She is grumpy and mean to classmates. Her body is very tired and cannot fight germs. She gets a cold.

Harmful Stress Can:

- increase the chance of heart disease.
- increase the chance of cancer.
- cause headaches.
- cause stomachaches.
- increase the chance of getting colds and flu.
- make you grumpy.

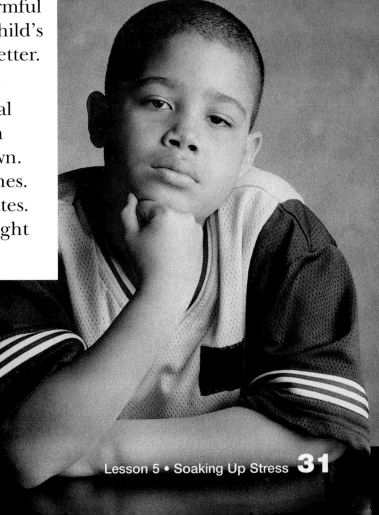

How Can I Control Harmful Stress?

There are ways to control harmful stress. There are ways to bounce back from hard times.

Talk about harmful stress with your parents, guardian, or another adult. Tell what causes you harmful stress. Suppose you do not know the cause. They can help you find the cause. Discuss what to do about harmful stress. They can suggest actions.

Ask your friends for support. Tell your friends you have harmful stress. They can help you bounce back. They can cheer you up. They can plan fun things to do to get your mind off hard times.

Write a plan for your day and check off what you complete. When you feel harmful stress, it can be hard to get things done. A plan helps you look at one thing at a time. You feel good each time one thing is done and checked off your list.

Get plenty of physical activity. Physical activity helps lessen harmful stress. It uses up the sugar in your blood. It helps blood flow to the brain so you can think clearly. Physical activity causes your body to make substances that make your mood better. **Beta-endorphins** (BAY·tuh·en·DOR·fuhns) are substances that make you feel good.

Get enough rest and sleep. Harmful stress makes you tired. You want to think clearly. Your body needs rest and sleep to be able to fight germs.

Eat healthful meals and snacks. Eat citrus fruits and drink juices to get vitamin C. Some health experts believe vitamin C helps your body fight germs.

Stress Adds Up

Life Skill

• **I will have a plan for stress.**

Materials: Colored paper, notebook paper, pencil, stapler

Directions: Complete the following activity to add up the stress you have in one week.

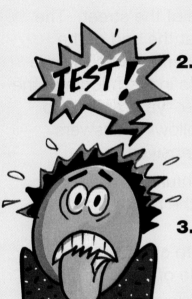

1. **Make a list of things that cause harmful stress.** You might include a disagreement with a friend or a test.

2. **Make a stress diary.** Use a sheet of colored paper for the front and back covers. Write "Stress Diary" on the front cover. Put seven sheets of notebook paper in your diary. Write a day of the week at the top of each sheet of notebook paper. Staple your stress diary together.

3. **Fill in your stress diary each day for a week.** Write down the things that cause you stress. Write what you did about them.

4. **Share your stress diary with your parents or guardian.**

Activity

Lesson 5

Review

Vocabulary

Write a separate sentence using each vocabulary word listed on page 28.

Health Content

1. What are kinds of stressors? **page 29**
2. What body changes does stress cause? **page 29**
3. What is healthful stress? **page 30**
4. What is harmful stress? **page 31**
5. How can you control harmful stress? **page 32**

Unit 1 Review

Health Content

1. What are the three parts of total health? **Lesson 1 page 6**

2. What are four steps to make a health behavior contract? **Lesson 1 page 8**

3. What can happen if you break rules? **Lesson 2 page 12**

4. What can you use when you need to say NO? **Lesson 2 page 14**

5. How might you describe friends who have good character? **Lesson 3 page 18**

6. What does it mean to "pay forward" for a mistake? **Lesson 3 page 19**

7. What is television addiction? **Lesson 4 page 24**

8. What are three things to put in an I-message? **Lesson 4 page 26**

9. How are healthful stress and harmful stress different? **Lesson 5 pages 30–31**

10. How does physical activity help control stress? **Lesson 5 page 32**

Guidelines for Making Responsible Decisions™

You and a friend are walking down a busy street. You need to be on the other side of the street. The crosswalk is at the end of the block. Your friend wants to save time and cross in the middle of the block. Answer "yes" or "no" to each of the following answers. Explain each answer.

1. Is it healthful to cross the street in the middle of the block?

2. Is it safe to cross the street in the middle of the block?

3. Do you follow rules and laws if you cross the street in the middle of the block?

4. Do you show respect for yourself and others if you cross the street in the middle of the block?

5. Do you follow your family's guidelines if you cross the street in the middle of the block?

6. Do you show good character if you cross the street in the middle of the block?

What is the responsible decision to make?

Vocabulary

Number a sheet of paper from 1–10. Read each definition. Next to each number on your sheet of paper, write the vocabulary word that matches the definition.

stressor	healthful stress
mood	addiction
good character	willpower
resistance skills	life skill
health behavior contract	rule

1. Ways to say NO to wrong decisions. **Lesson 2**
2. A healthful action you practice now and for the rest of your life. **Lesson 1**
3. Anything that causes stress. **Lesson 5**
4. A guide to help you do the right thing. **Lesson 2**
5. Stress that helps you perform well and stay healthy. **Lesson 5**
6. Telling the truth, showing respect, and being fair. **Lesson 2**
7. The way you feel at certain times. **Lesson 4**
8. The strength you need to do the right thing. **Lesson 3**
9. Letting a drug or habit control you. **Lesson 4**
10. A written plan to help you practice a life skill. **Lesson 1**

Health Literacy

Effective Communication

Think about the last time you were angry. Write an I-message to express your angry feelings.

Self-Directed Learning

Find an article or story about stress. Read the article or story. Write a few sentences to tell what you learned.

Critical Thinking

Why do you need good character? Answer the question on a separate sheet of paper.

Responsible Citizenship

A pledge is a promise to do something. Write a six-line pledge about character. Teach your classmates the pledge that you write.

Family Involvement

Ask your parents or guardian to play a game to make your memory better. You might play Concentration or another card game. You might choose a board game. You might use flash cards.

Unit 2

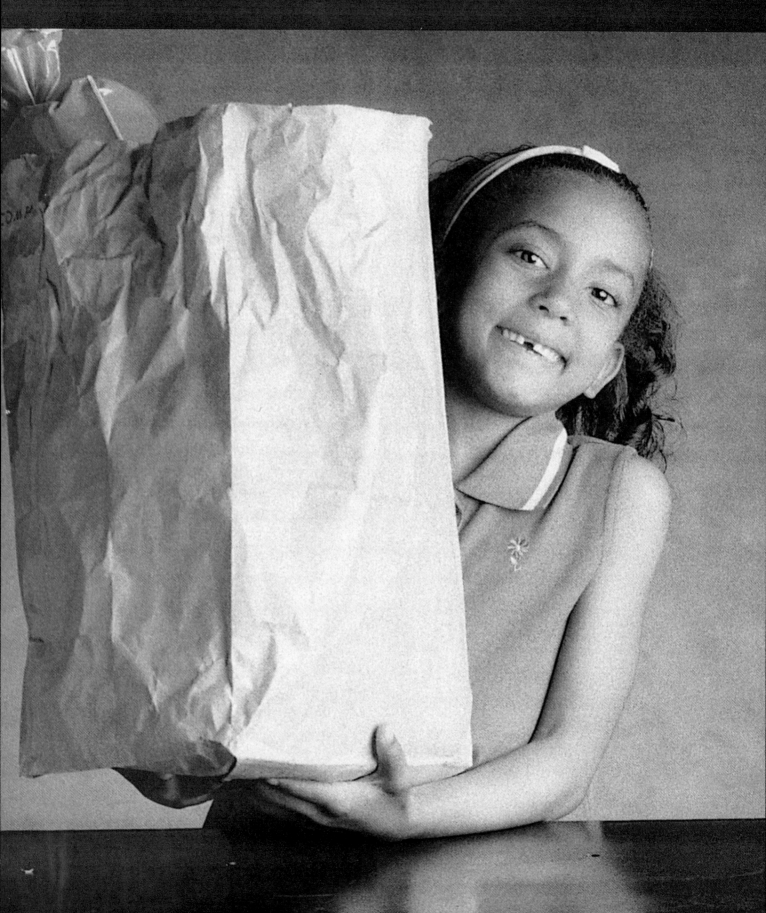

Family and
Social Health

Lesson 6
Respect for All

Lesson 7
Patch Up Disagreements

Lesson 8
Wanted: True Friends

Lesson 9
Reach Out to Family

Respect for All

Vocabulary

respect: thinking highly of someone.

self-respect: thinking highly of yourself.

set limits: to be clear as to what is OK and what is not OK with you.

honest talk: saying exactly how you feel.

doormat: a person whom other people walk all over.

Life Skill

- I will show respect for all people.

Respect is thinking highly of someone. You need to show respect for other people. You need to show respect for yourself. Other people need to show respect for you. Showing respect and getting respect is part of family and social health.

The Lesson Objectives

- Tell how to show respect for others.
- List ways you can tell if someone does not show respect for you.
- Tell why you need to show respect for yourself.
- Discuss what to do if someone does not show respect for you.

How Can I Show Respect for Others?

Do not ask other people to do anything wrong. You do not want someone you care about to get into trouble. You do not want this person to have bad character. You want the best for the person.

Respect the family guidelines of other people. Your friends must follow their family guidelines. Help them to do so. Suppose a friend is not allowed to ride her bike in the street. Do not suggest that she does. Remind her of her family's guidelines.

Do not choose actions that might harm the health of others. Show you think highly of others by helping them stay healthy. Suppose you have friends over after school. A friend has a health condition and cannot have sugar. Do not offer the friend a candy bar. Offer the friend a snack he can eat.

Do not choose actions that risk the safety of others. Suppose you are biking in a park where other people walk and run. Stay in the lane marked for biking. Do not get into another lane. If you do, you might crash into people who are walking or running. Show respect by keeping them safe.

Do not harm others with violence. *Violence* is harm done to yourself, others, or property. Do not kick, bite, push, or punch someone. Do not take things that do not belong to you or harm property.

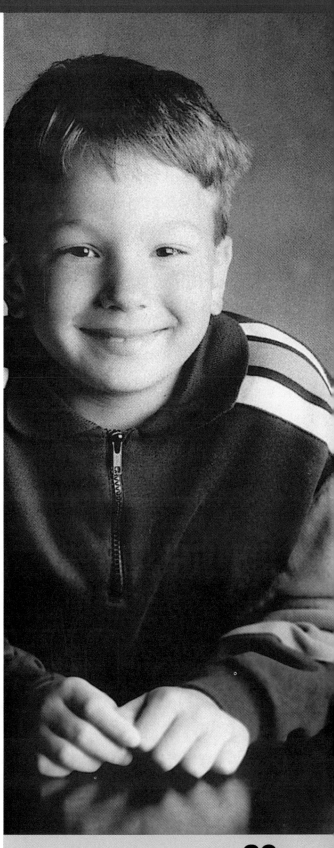

What Can I Do If Someone Does Not Show Respect for Me?

Check out your self-respect. This is the first thing to do. **Self-respect** is thinking highly of yourself. When you have self-respect, you take good care of yourself. Suppose you do not treat yourself well. Maybe you put down yourself. Other people might see that you treat yourself badly and think it is OK if they do.

Set limits for the actions of other people. To **set limits** is to be clear as to what is OK and what is not OK with you. For example, it is OK if someone disagrees with you. It is not OK if someone punches you over a disagreement.

Use honest talk with the person. Suppose someone does not show respect for you. The person does something that is not OK. For example, the person might grab something away from you. Use honest talk. **Honest talk** is saying exactly how you feel. You might say, "I do not like it when you grab something from me."

Ask the person to change the actions that do not show respect. You might say, "Please do not grab something away from me again."

Stay away from a person who will not change actions after you have talked.

A Person Does Not Respect You If He or She:

- asks you to do something wrong.
- tries to get you to break your family's guidelines.
- acts in ways that might harm your health.
- acts in ways that put your safety at risk.
- harms you with violence.

What Does It Mean to Act Like a Doormat?

A **doormat** is a person whom other people walk all over. Usually this person does not have self-respect. The person allows other people to treat him or her in unkind ways. What if this describes you? Talk to your parents or guardian or a counselor at school. Learn to think highly of yourself. Learn to set limits for the ways other people treat you.

I Get No Respect

Life Skill

• **I will show respect for all people.**

Materials: Large sheet of poster paper, marker

Directions: Complete this activity to see what it is like to get no respect.

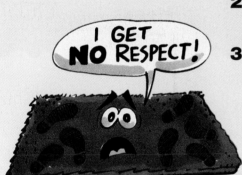

1. Someone must write "I get no respect" on the poster paper.

2. Tape the poster paper to the floor to be a doormat.

3. Classmates will take a turn walking on the poster paper. Suppose it is your turn. Walk on the poster paper. Say a way a person might give you no respect. For example, you might say, "I get no respect when someone pushes me." And then add, "and I do not like it." All classmates take a turn.

Activity

Lesson 6

Review

Vocabulary

Write a separate sentence using each vocabulary word listed on page 38.

Health Content

1. How can you show respect for others? **page 39**

2. What are ways you know if someone does not respect you? **page 40**

3. Why do you need self-respect? **page 40**

4. What can you do if someone does not show respect for you? **page 40**

5. What does it mean to act like a doormat? **page 40**

Lesson 7

Patch Up Disagreements

Vocabulary

conflict: a disagreement.

gossip: saying unkind things about a person.

coward: a person who is not strong inside.

fight: a struggle between two or more people.

weapon: an object used to harm someone.

Life Skill

• I will settle conflict in healthful ways.

A **conflict** is a disagreement. Everyone has disagreements. You can learn ways to patch up disagreements. You can patch up disagreements without saying unkind words about someone. You can patch up disagreements without trying to frighten or hurt someone. You can patch up a disagreement without fighting.

The Lesson Objectives

• Discuss ways to be fair.

• Tell why it is wrong to gossip.

• Tell what to do if someone gossips about you.

• Discuss what to do about a bully.

• Discuss what to do if someone wants you to fight.

How Can I Be Fair?

Conflict can happen when a person is not fair. You can keep conflict from happening. There are ways to be fair.

Do not take things that belong to someone else. Suppose a classmate is not looking. You take your classmate's cookie at lunch. You put it in your bag to eat later. Your classmate can find out and get angry. Then you have a conflict.

Do not use things or borrow things without asking. Suppose you take a game that belongs to your sister. She looks for the game and cannot find it. She finds out you took it without asking. She is angry. Then you have a conflict.

Do not take more than your share of something. Suppose your older sister makes brownies for the family. The plate of brownies is sitting out. You eat most of the brownies off the plate. Your brother does not get any. Then you have a conflict.

Take turns. Suppose you play ball with friends. You keep the ball most of the time. Your friends get tired of you being a ball hog. Then you have a conflict.

Play by the rules. Suppose you swim at a pool. There is a rule against dunking. You dunk your friend. Your friend gets angry. Then you have a conflict.

It's Fairly Simple

I've been waiting here
in line.

But to you, that's just
NOT fine.

You push and shove
to get ahead.

"I don't think that's
fair," I said.

Why can't you just
wait like me?

And be as patient
as you can be.

But if you have
an emergency.

I'll let you get ahead
of me.

Sometimes things
just do arise.

And then I get caught
by surprise.

Share your feelings
and explain to me.

And I'll be fair, just
wait and see.

Why Is It Wrong to Gossip?

Conflict can happen if you gossip. **Gossip** is saying unkind things about a person. When people gossip, they say unkind things about a person to another person.

Other people will not trust you if you gossip. Suppose your friend tells you something that upsets her. You tell some of your classmates what she said. She will not trust you.

Other people will have hurt feelings if you gossip about them. Suppose your friend gets a haircut. You make fun of the friend's haircut to a classmate. Your friend finds out and is hurt.

Other people can get angry and try to get even. Suppose you say something that is not true about a person. The person finds out and gets angry. The person might say things that are untrue about you.

Other people will think you are a coward. A **coward** is a person who is not strong inside. The person is not strong enough to tell you the truth. Suppose your friend does something you do not like. You tell other people what your friend did. You do this instead of telling your friend. Your friend thinks you are a coward.

What to Do If Someone Gossips About You

- Set limits. Be clear that you do not want anyone to gossip about you.

- Use honest talk. Stand up for yourself. Say exactly how you feel. You might feel angry or hurt.

- Ask the person to stop saying gossip about you.

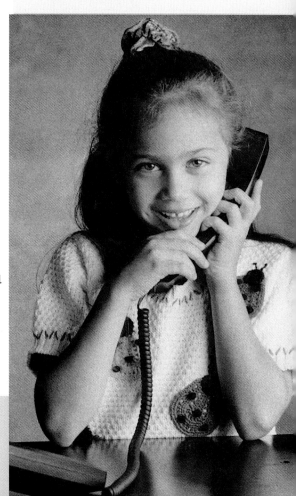

What Can I Do About a Bully?

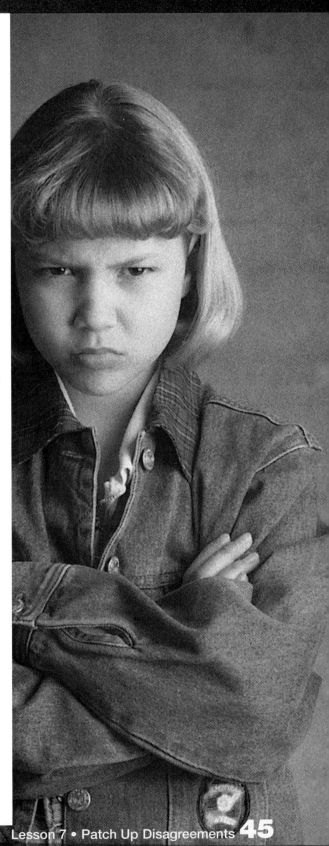

Conflict can happen if someone is a bully. A *bully* is a person who tries to frighten or hurt someone who is younger or smaller. Suppose an older boy tells you to give him a dime or you cannot get on the school bus. He is acting like a bully.

Never act like a bully. Other people will not want to be around you. They will not trust you. Other people can get angry. If they get a chance, they might try to get even. These are actions you can take around a bully.

Ask the bully to stop trying to frighten or hurt you. Use honest talk. Say exactly how you feel. You might say, "I do not like it when you try to push me around. I do not like it when you try to take things from me."

Get away from the bully. Do not get near a bully who tries to hurt you. Stay away if the bully tries to kick or punch you. Run as fast as you can. Scream as loud as you can.

Ask your parent, guardian, or other trusted adult for help. A bully can be very mean. An adult might need to keep you safe. An adult might need to contact the parents or guardian of the bully. An adult might need to contact someone at your school or the police. A bully needs the help of responsible adults.

What Can I Do If Someone Wants Me to Fight?

A **fight** is a struggle between two or more people. The fight might be with words. Two or more people might scream, shout, and call each other names. They might use put-downs. A fight might be physical. Two or more people might punch, kick, shove or bite.

People might use weapons in a fight. A **weapon** is an object used to harm someone. A knive, razor, or gun might be used to harm someone. A brick, broom, or belt might be used to harm someone.

Suppose someone wants to fight with you. This is never the way to deal with conflict. You and the other person can get hurt.

What to Do If Someone Wants to Fight.

- Say you do not want to fight.
- Say you were wrong if you did something wrong. Offer to make up for what you did.
- Wait until you are calm and talk things out.
- Get away from a situation if the person tries to harm you.
- Ask a parent, guardian, or other adult for help.

Drinking and Fighting

Drinking alcohol can change how a person reasons. It can make feelings strong. A person who is angry can get more angry. This person is more likely to start a fight. Do not drink alcohol. Stay away from an angry person who has been drinking.

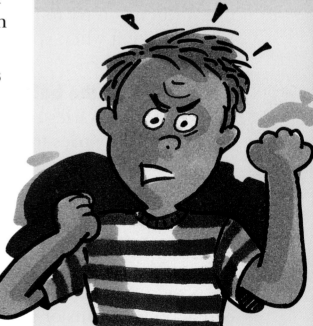

What Happens If I Repeat It?

Life Skill

- I will settle conflict in healthful ways.

Materials: None

Directions: Complete this activity to learn what can happen if you gossip.

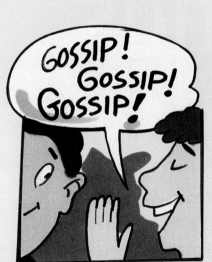

1. **Your teacher will write gossip about a person who is not real.** Your teacher will not let you see the gossip he or she wrote.

2. **Your teacher will whisper the gossip to one of your classmates.** This classmate will whisper the gossip to another classmate. Keep going until all classmates have heard the gossip.

3. **The last classmate to hear the gossip repeats it to the class.** Does it match what the teacher wrote?

Activity

Lesson 7

Review

Vocabulary

Write a separate sentence using each vocabulary word listed on page 42.

Health Content

1. What are ways to be fair? **page 43**

2. Why is it wrong to gossip? **page 44**

3. What might you do if someone gossips about you? **page 44**

4. What can you do about a bully? **page 45**

5. What can you do if someone wants you to fight? **page 46**

Wanted: True Friends

Vocabulary

true friend: a friend whose actions are responsible and caring.

skill: something you do that takes practice.

friend who has special needs: a friend who has needs that are different from others.

life skill: a healthful action you learn and practice for life.

health behavior contract: a written plan to help you practice a life skill.

Life Skills

- I will work to have healthful friendships.
- I will encourage other people to take care of their health.

A **true friend** is a friend whose actions are responsible and caring. True friends make responsible decisions together. True friends help each other practice life skills. Some true friends have special needs. It is worth making and keeping true friends.

The Lesson Objectives

- Tell why you need true friends.
- Tell ways to make a true friend.
- Explain how friends can make responsible decisions.
- Explain how friends can help each other practice life skills.

Why Do I Need True Friends?

True friends teach you how to get along with others. You practice being a true friend. You practice working out disagreements. You learn how much effort it takes to have healthful relationships.

True friends help you when you feel stress. Suppose your pet dies. You feel down in the dumps. Your true friends care that you are sad. They listen when you talk about your sad feelings.

True friends enjoy physical activities with you. After school and on weekends, you have extra time. True friends can spend time with you. You might skate, ski, or jump rope. You get healthy and have fun at the same time.

True friends listen to your ideas. An idea is a thought or belief. You are learning a lot right now. You have many new thoughts. As you learn facts, you form beliefs. You test out your ideas on friends.

True friends protect you from harm. Suppose you think about making a wrong decision. True friends warn you of the bad outcomes that can happen. They remind you of your family's guidelines. They remind you of school rules.

True friends give you the chance to show that you are a caring person. Suppose a true friend has stress. You support your true friend. As a result, you feel good about yourself.

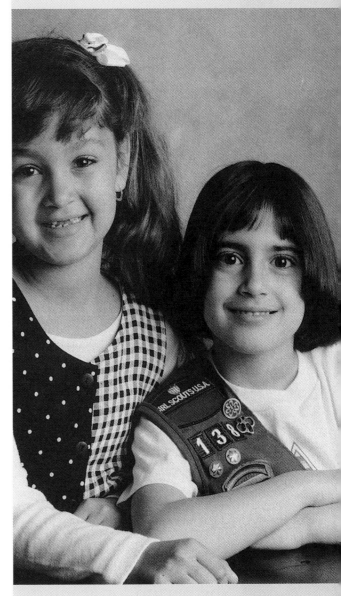

How Can I Make a True Friend?

A **skill** is something you do that takes practice. One skill is making a true friend.

Think about places to meet someone who might become a true friend.

There might be someone at school or in your neighborhood. Suppose you join a club or sports team. There might be children you do not know.

Get permission from your parents or guardian to get together with someone.

Your parents or guardian want to know with whom you spend time. Tell them you want to get together with someone.

Make plans to get together.
You might want to get together with other children at first. Talk about what you will do. Plan an activity you both enjoy. Feel OK about yourself if the person says NO.

Be certain that the person is caring and responsible.
It takes time to make a true friend. You must spend time wisely. Check out what the person is like. Does the person make responsible decisions? Follow family guidelines? Choose healthful behaviors? Show respect for you?

Put time and effort into being a true friend.
To make a true friend, you must be a true friend. Treat the person well. Be responsible and caring. Do not take the person for granted. With hard work, you can make a true friend.

How Can I Be a True Friend to a Person Who Has Special Needs?

A **friend who has special needs** is a friend who has needs that are different from others. You might make friends with a person who uses a wheelchair. Your friend has special needs. Your friend might use a ramp to enter a building. Your friend might play basketball or baseball while he or she is in a wheelchair. You can be a true friend to a person who has special needs.

- Talk about ways to meet the special needs your friend has.

- Plan activities that your friend can do with you.

- Know that most of your needs—for caring and support—are the same.

How Can Friends Make Responsible Decisions?

When you are with friends, you must make responsible decisions. Here are three rules to help you make responsible decisions with friends.

Use the Guidelines for Making Responsible Decisions™. Suppose you and a friend must make a decision. You disagree about what to do. Before you decide, use the six questions in the Guidelines.

Stop your friend if he or she is about to make a wrong decision. Suppose you and a friend are walking to a movie. You are going to be late. He puts his thumb out to hitchhike. Remind your friend of the Guidelines. It is not safe for him to hitchhike. It is not legal for him to hitchhike. His parents or guardian do not want him to hitchhike. You help protect him from danger.

Do not go along with a friend's wrong decisions. Suppose your friend still keeps his thumb up. He is going to make a wrong decision. Do not go along with your friend's wrong decision. Do not put your thumb up to hitchhike. Do not get into the car with someone you do not know. When a friend makes a wrong decision, protect yourself from harm. Get out of the situation. Call your parents or guardian.

Friends Use the Guidelines for Making Responsible Decisions™

They ask:

1. Is it healthful to_____?
2. Is it safe to _____?
3. Do we follow rules and laws if we _____?
4. Do we show respect for ourselves and others if we _____?
5. Do we both follow our family's guidelines if we _____?
6. Do we show good character if we _____?

How Can Friends Practice Life Skills Together?

A **life skill** is a healthful action you learn and practice for life. Here are two ways friends can practice life skills together.

Help each other make a health behavior contract. A **health behavior contract** is a written plan to help you practice a life skill. Suppose you and a friend want to change how you eat. Both of you eat snacks with lots of sugar and salt. You want to help each other practice this life skill: "I will eat healthful meals and snacks." Each of you can make your own health behavior contract.

Take turns choosing a healthful behavior to do after school or on weekends. Suppose it is your turn to choose. You might suggest ice skating or taking a walk. Then you and your friend get plenty of physical activity.

Suppose its your friend's turn to choose. Your friend might suggest going to the library to find a book. Then you and a friend choose to keep your minds healthy.

Four Steps to Make a Health Behavior Contract

1. Write the life skill you want to practice.

2. Tell how the life skill helps you to be healthy.

3. Write what you plan to do.

4. Tell what happened when you tried the plan.

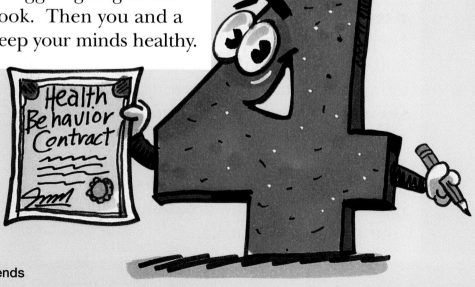

Use... Guidelines for Making Responsible Decisions™

Situation:

You are with a friend at a fast food restaurant. A woman sits down at the table next to yours. She has French fries, a chicken sandwich, and soda. She gets up to go to the restroom. Your friend says, "Let's take her food and get out of here."

Response:

Answer "yes" or "no" to each of the following questions. Explain each answer.

1. Is it healthful to take her lunch?
2. Is it safe to take her lunch?
3. Do you follow rules and laws if you take her lunch?
4. Do you show respect for yourself and the woman if you take her lunch?
5. Do you follow your family's guidelines if you take her lunch?
6. Do you show good character if you take her lunch?

What is the responsible decision to make?

Lesson 8

Review

Vocabulary

Write a separate sentence using each vocabulary word listed on page 48.

Health Content

1. Why do you need to have true friends? **page 49**
2. What are steps to take to make a true friend? **page 50**
3. How can you be a true friend to a person who has special needs? **page 50**
4. What are three rules to help you make responsible decisions with friends? **page 51**
5. What are two ways friends can practice life skills together? **page 52**

Reach Out to Family

Vocabulary

family: a group of people who are related.

message: words or body movements used to say something to another person.

memory: something from the past that you remember.

family value: the importance of something to your family.

adopt: to bring a child from other parents into your family.

Life Skills

- I will work to have healthful family relationships.
- I will adjust to family changes in healthful ways.

A **family** is a group of people who are related. There are many kinds of families. Some families are large while others are small. In some families, all the members live in the same city or state. In other families, family members live far apart.

The Lesson Objectives

- Tell the special names for each person who belongs to a family.
- Discuss ways families are alike.
- Explain how to be a loving family member.
- Explain how a family changes when there is a new baby or child.
- Explain how a family changes if parents divorce or remarry.

Who Belongs to a Family?

There are special names for each person in a family. These names show how people are related to each other.

Mother: female parent of a child.

Father: male parent of a child.

Daughter: female child. A girl or woman is the daughter of her mother and father.

Son: male child. A boy or man is the son of his mother and father.

Brother: boy or man having the same parents as another person.

Sister: girl or woman having the same parents as another person.

Grandmother: mother of a person's mother or father.

Grandfather: father of a person's mother or father.

Granddaughter: daughter of a person's son or daughter.

Grandson: son of a person's son or daughter.

Aunt: sister of a person's mother or father. The wife of a person's uncle.

Uncle: brother of a person's mother or father. The husband of a person's aunt.

Cousin: son or daughter of an aunt or uncle.

Brother-in-law: brother of a person's husband or wife. The husband of a sister.

Sister-in-law: sister of a person's husband or wife. The wife of a brother.

Family Members from Remarriage

To *remarry* means to get married again. A husband and wife might get a divorce. A *divorce* is a legal way to end a marriage. If either one remarries, there are new family members. A husband or wife might die. The living partner might remarry.

Stepfather: man married to someone's mother after the divorce or death of the real father.

Stepmother: woman married to someone's father after the divorce or death of the real mother.

Stepson: son of a person's husband or wife from another marriage.

Stepdaughter: daughter of a person's second husband or wife.

Stepbrother: son of a person's stepmother or stepfather.

Stepsister: daughter of a person's stepmother or stepfather.

How Are Families Alike?

Messages are sent in families. A **message** is words or body movements used to say something to another person. There are many messages sent between family members. A smile or frown is a message. A hug is a message.

Suppose you write a note to your mother. The note says, "I love you." You have sent a loving message to your mother.

Some messages in families show concern, love, and understanding. These messages help family members know they are loved by other family members.

In some families, messages between family members cause unhappiness. Family members yell and scream. They might not talk at all. They might use put-downs and say mean things. These messages do not help family members feel loved.

- Set aside time to talk to family members.

- Give messages that show concern, love, and understanding.

- Do not use put-downs or yell and scream at family members.

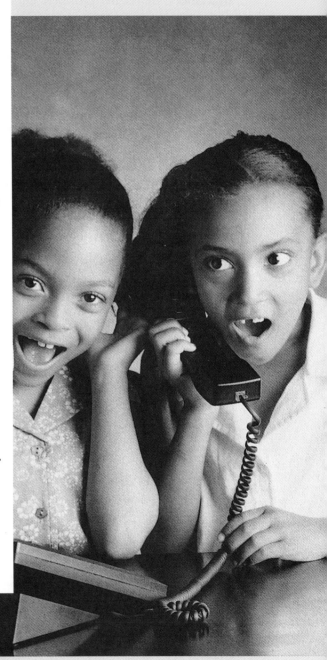

Memories are made in families. A **memory** is something from the past that you remember. All family members have memories. There are different kinds of memories. Suppose your family had a pet that was hit by a car. This is a sad family memory. Suppose your family took a vacation. The vacation was a happy family memory.

Family memories can last a long time. What you do today in your family becomes a memory tomorrow.

- Do something today to make a happy family memory.

- Talk to your parents or guardian about a memory that bothers you.

Values are learned in families. A **family value** is the importance of something to your family. Good health might be important to your parents or guardian. They want good health to be a family value. They do not let people smoke in your home or car. They buy healthful foods for your family.

When you learn what is right and wrong, you are learning values. Your family teaches you to tell the truth. They teach you to be fair. Values help you make choices.

- Ask your parents or guardian to tell you family values.

- Practice family values.

Why Keep a Family Album of Photos?

Many families keep an album of photos. They write about the photos. They say where they were and when. The family can look at the photos and talk about their memories.

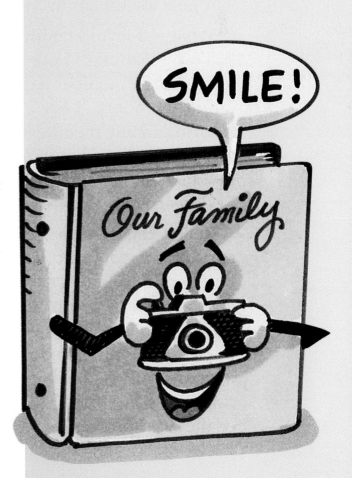

How Can I Be a Loving Family Member?

Have you ever found a four-leaf clover? A four-leaf clover is not easy to find. Being hard to find makes a four-leaf clover special. Some people will press a four-leaf clover between the pages of a book so they can keep it. They keep it with them for good luck.

The four-leaf clover in the margin tells what a loving family member is like. A loving family member is special. You can be a loving family member.

What is a loving family member? Love has two meanings. Love is a feeling. A loving family member feels love for other family members. Love also is an action. A loving family members acts in loving ways. To be a loving family member, you need loving feelings and loving actions. Let's learn about loving actions.

A loving family member shows respect for other family members. You show that you think other family members are worthy. You do not interrupt when they speak. You give them privacy when they need it. For example, you do not go into the bathroom when they are using it. You do not take something of theirs without asking. You do not talk back or say mean things.

Just Like a Four-Leaf Clover...

A loving family member is special.

A loving family member:

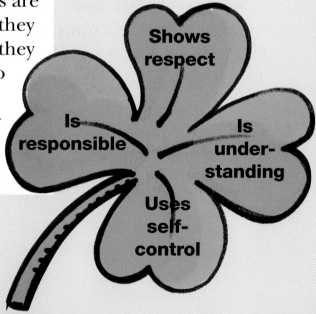

Shows respect

Is responsible

Is under-standing

Uses self-control

A loving family member is responsible.

Suppose you are responsible. Other family members can depend on you. They know you will do what you are supposed to do. Perhaps you have certain chores to do. A chore is a small job. You might set the table or take the trash out. You might help with the dishes. You get your chores done without being reminded.

A loving family member is understanding.

Suppose you are understanding. You care about how your actions affect other family members. Perhaps your mother has worked very hard today. You turn down the sound on the radio while she takes a nap. Perhaps your brother lost a baseball game. You give your brother a hug and tell him you are proud of him.

A loving family member uses self-control.

Self-control is being able to hold back from doing something you should not do. Suppose your parent or guardian says you can ride your bike to a friend's home. You are not allowed to stop anywhere else. On the way, you meet another friend. This friend wants you to stop for an ice cream cone. You would really like to have an ice cream cone. But you hold back. You use self-control and do not have the ice cream. You keep yourself from doing something you should not do.

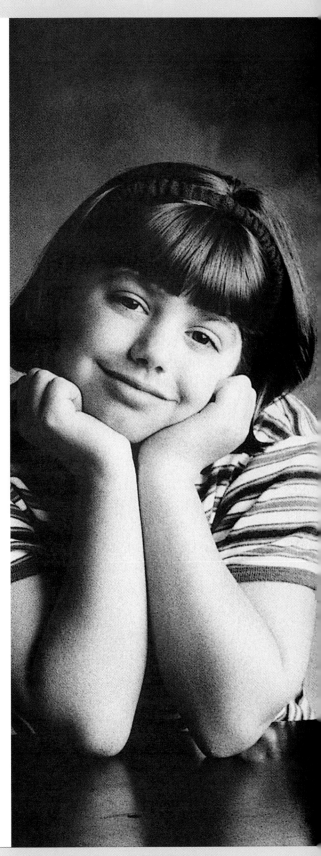

How Might Having or Adopting a Baby or Child Change a Family?

Many changes take place in a family when a baby is born. Some of these changes are easy to accept. You might enjoy holding a baby. Showing a new baby to friends can be fun.

Other changes can be more difficult to accept. A new baby might cry often. A new baby must be cared for and fed often. This takes a lot of time.

The other children in a family might wish the baby did not take so much of the parents' time. The other children might want more attention.

A family can talk about these changes. Children can talk about their feelings. Their parents' can tell the children how important they are.

A family might choose to adopt a child. To **adopt** is to bring a child from other parents into your family. Some children are adopted shortly after they are born. Some children are adopted when they are older.

There are changes when a child is adopted. If the child is a baby, other children in the family learn about caring for a baby. If the adopted child is older, there are changes, too. The adopted child and other children must learn to understand each other.

Other Family Changes

There can be family changes if parents get a divorce or remarry. Children might have questions about changes. They can ask their parents with whom they will live. They can find out when they will see each parent. Children might have many feelings. They might feel sad. They might feel angry. They might feel guilty. To feel guilty is to think you made something happen. Children do not cause parents to divorce. Children need to share their feelings with their parents. If a parent remarries, there are more changes. There might be stepbrothers or stepsisters. There might be new rules. It takes time to get used to the changes. Talking helps.

Coupons for Chores

Life Skill

- I will work to have healthful family relationships.

Materials: Sample coupons, scissors, markers, crayons, or pen

Directions: A coupon is a ticket you can exchange for something. A *chore* is a small job. Plan to give your parents or guardian coupons which show chores you will do.

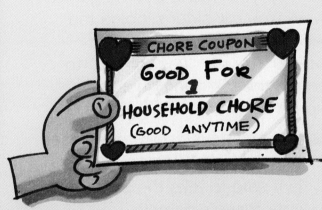

1. **Look at the sample coupons.**

2. **Make a coupon for five chores you can do at home.**

3. **Give the five chore coupons to your parents or guardian.** Tell them they can use them at any time.

Activity

Lesson 9

Review

Vocabulary

Write a separate sentence using each vocabulary word listed on page 54.

Health Content

1. What are the names of five people who belong to a family? **page 55**

2. What are three ways families are alike? **pages 56–57**

3. What are four ways to be a loving family member? **pages 58–59**

4. How might having or adopting a baby or child change a family? **page 60**

5. How might parents' divorce or remarriage change a family? **page 60**

Unit 2 Review

Health Content

1. What are ways to show respect for others? **Lesson 6 page 39**

2. What is honest talk? **Lesson 6 page 40**

3. How can you be fair to others? **Lesson 7 page 43**

4. Why is it wrong to gossip? **Lesson 7 page 44**

5. What can you do if someone gossips about you? **Lesson 7 page 44**

6. Why do you need true friends? **Lesson 8 page 49**

7. How can you be a true friend to a person who has special needs? **Lesson 8 page 50**

8. What is a stepmother? Stepfather? **Lesson 9 page 55**

9. How can you work on the messages you give family members? **Lesson 9 page 56**

10. What are four actions to show you are a loving family member? **Lesson 9 pages 58–59**

Guidelines for Making Responsible Decisions™

You play a game at a friend's house. You have the same game at home but you do not have one of the pieces. When you are done, you help your friend put the game away. You consider slipping the piece you are missing into your pocket. Answer "yes" or "no" to each of the following questions. Explain each answer.

1. Is it healthful to take the piece of your friend's game?

2. Is it safe to take the piece of your friend's game?

3. Do you follow rules and laws if you take the piece of your friend's game?

4. Do you show respect for yourself and others if you take the piece of your friend's game?

5. Do you follow your family's guidelines if you take the piece of your friend's game?

6. Do you show good character if you take the piece of your friend's game?

What is the responsible decision to make?

Vocabulary

Number a sheet of paper from 1–10. Read each definition. Next to each number on your sheet of paper, write the vocabulary word that matches the definition.

self-respect	coward
memory	conflict
adopt	respect
true friend	family value
friend who has special needs	gossip

1. A disagreement. **Lesson 7**
2. The importance of something to your family. **Lesson 9**
3. Thinking highly of someone. **Lesson 6**
4. Saying unkind things about a person. **Lesson 7**
5. To bring a child from other parents into your family. **Lesson 9**
6. Thinking highly of yourself. **Lesson 6**
7. A friend who has needs that are different from others. **Lesson 8**
8. A friend whose actions are responsible and caring. **Lesson 8**
9. Something from the past that you remember. **Lesson 9**
10. A person who is not strong inside. **Lesson 7**

Health Literacy

Effective Communication

Make a greeting card for a friend. The card should tell your friend why he or she is special to you.

Self-Directed Learning

Make a word search using the names of family members in Lesson 9. Give your word search to a classmate.

Critical Thinking

What might happen if you tell gossip about a true friend? Answer the question on a separate sheet of paper.

Responsible Citizenship

Suppose someone at your school has a weapon. Name two adults at your school you might tell.

Family Involvement

Ask your parents or guardian to show you at least three family photos. Discuss the family memories that go with the three photos.

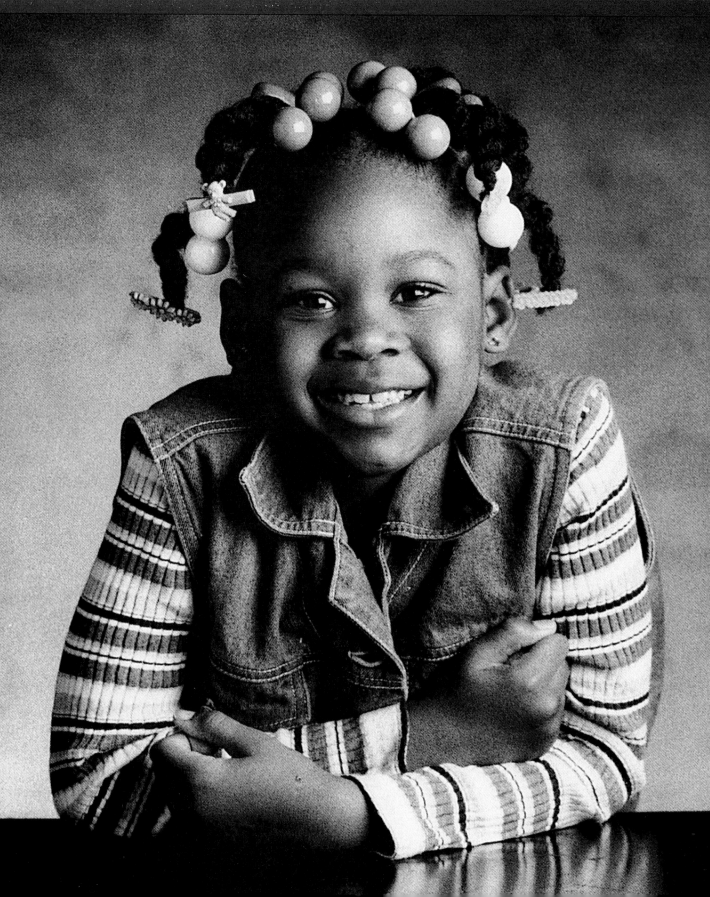

Growth and Development

All About Body Systems

Vocabulary

A list of body system vocabulary is on page 67.

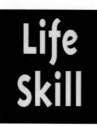
Life Skill

- **I will care for my body systems.**

Your body is made up of many body systems. You can learn what the parts of each system do. You can learn ways to take care of each body system.

The Lesson Objectives

- Tell what the parts of the skeletal system do.
- Tell what the parts of the muscular system do.
- Tell what the parts of the nervous system do.
- Tell what the parts of the digestive system do.
- Tell what the parts of the circulatory system do.
- Tell what the parts of the respiratory system do.

What Is a Body System?

Each of your body parts is made of cells. A *cell* is the smallest living part of a person's body. Most cells are so small they can be seen only with a microscope.

Your body has many types of cells. Some types include skin cells, blood cells, muscle cells, and bone cells. Each type of cell does a special kind of work.

Your body makes new cells every day. New cells are important for your growth. New cells take the places of cells that die. You grow because your body makes new cells faster than old cells die.

Some cells in the body are alike. Cells that are alike form tissues. A *tissue* (TI·shoo) is a group of cells that work together to do a special job. Muscle is an example of a tissue. Muscle is made of cells that are alike.

An *organ* is a body part made of different kinds of tissues. Your heart is an organ. It is made of tissues that work together to pump blood throughout your body. Your eyes and ears also are organs.

A *body system* is a group of organs that work together to do a certain job. Your heart, blood, and blood vessels form a body system that helps blood travel to all cells in your body.

Body System Vocabulary

- The **skeletal system** is the group of bones in your body.

- The **muscular system** is the system made up of all the muscles in your body.

- The **nervous system** is made of organs that control all your body actions.

- The **digestive system** is made up of organs that help your body use food.

- The **circulatory system** is made up of organs that move blood throughout your body.

- The **respiratory system** is made up of organs that help you use the air you breathe.

What Do the Parts of the Skeletal System Do?

The **skeletal** (SKE·luh·tuhl) **system** is the group of bones in your body. Your skeletal system gives your body support and shape. Along with your muscles, your skeletal system helps you move.

Your skull Your *skull* is the bones on your head and the bones of your face. Your skull is made up of eight different bones. Your skull covers and protects your brain.

Your ribs Your *ribs* are the bones that cover and protect your heart and lungs. Your ribs also help support your shoulders and arms. You have 12 pairs of ribs.

Your vertebrae Your *vertebrae* (VUHR·tuh·bray) are 26 bones that make up your spine, or backbone. Your spine supports your body and your head. It protects your spinal cord. Your spinal cord is a long column of nerve cells that attaches to your brain. It runs down your back inside your spine. Your vertebrae let you bend in many directions.

Your femurs Your *femurs* (FEE·muhrz) are your thigh bones. They are the largest and strongest bones in your body. Your femurs support the weight of your upper body.

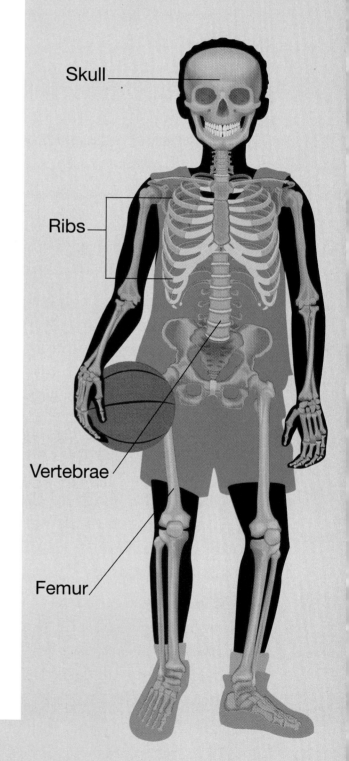

Skull

Ribs

Vertebrae

Femur

Physical activity makes your bones thicker. Choose activities in which you carry your own weight. Walking and running are good choices. Dancing also makes your bones thicker. You also might play sports in which you run. Soccer, baseball, and hockey are examples. In-line skating and ice skating make bones thicker. Doing push-ups and pull-ups makes bones thicker, too. Thick bones are less likely to break.

Calcium, phosphorus, and vitamin D make your bones strong. Calcium and phosphorus are minerals. They make bones strong. Vitamin D makes bones strong, too. Foods from the milk group have calcium, phosphorus and vitamin D in them. Milk, cheese, and yogurt are good choices. Green leafy vegetables and beans have calcium in them. Beans also have phosphorus in them. Strong bones give your body better support.

Good posture allows your bones to support your body in the right way. *Posture* (PAHS·chuhr) is the way you hold your body as you sit, stand, and move. When you have good posture, you sit and stand straight. You hold your head up and keep your shoulders back. Good posture keeps your back from hurting.

What Do Joints Do?

A *joint* is the place where bones meet. Joints help you bend and move. The joint at your knee helps you bend your leg. The joint at your arm helps you bend your arm.

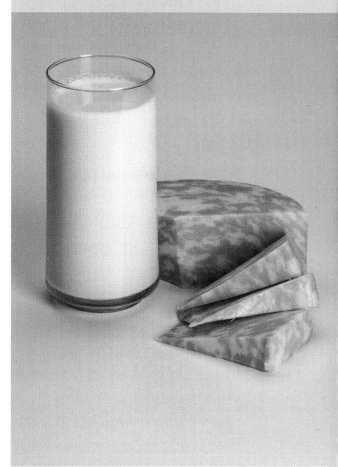

What Do the Parts of the Muscular System Do?

Your **muscular** (MUHS·kyuh·luhr) **system** is the system made up of all the muscles in your body. A *muscle* (MUH·suhl) is a tissue that allows your body to move. Some muscles are attached to bones. They work together to help you move.

Your arm muscles Your arm muscles help you lift things over your head. They help you carry things. Your arm muscles help you pull open a door. They help you push your chair toward the table. Your arm muscles help you throw and catch a ball.

Your thigh muscles Your thigh muscles are muscles that are in the upper legs. Your thigh muscles move your leg forward and backward at the hip and knee. These muscles help you walk.

Your calf muscles Your calf muscles are muscles in the back of your lower leg. Your calf muscles bend your leg at the ankle. Strong calf muscles are needed for many sports. You use calf muscles when you run, walk, ski, skate, and bike.

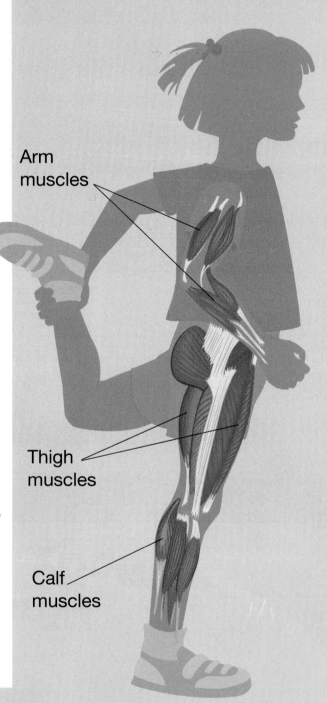

Arm muscles

Thigh muscles

Calf muscles

Physical activity makes your muscles stronger. Regular physical activity makes the muscles thicker. Then muscles are stronger. They can help you lift, pull, push, and kick with force. They can keep working without tiring. Then you can use your muscles for a longer time. For example, you can run a mile without your leg muscles tiring. Your heart muscle is strong. You can climb stairs without getting out of breath. Choose many kinds of physical activities. Walk, run, and bike. Play sports like baseball and soccer. Enjoy dancing.

Stretching exercises keep your muscles flexible. *Flexibility* (flek·suh·BI·luh·tee) is the ability to bend and move easily. You should do stretching exercises at least two to three times a week. Stretch a muscle until you feel a slight pull. Then hold the stretch until you count to fifteen. Always stretch your muscles before a hard workout. Do some stretches after you work out, too.

Calcium and magnesium help muscles work well. Calcium and magnesium are minerals. Foods from the milk group have calcium in them. Choose milk, cheese, and yogurt for calcium. Eat green leafy vegetables for calcium and magnesium. Eat nuts, beans, cereals, breads, and seafood for magnesium.

How Can I Stretch Leg Muscles?

Stand in front of a wall. Put your hands on the wall at the same height as your shoulders. Keep your arms straight. Put your right foot forward with your knee bent. Put your left leg back so the leg is straight. Try to keep your left foot flat on the floor. Feel the pull on your left calf muscle. Hold the stretch until you count to fifteen. Switch legs and stretch your right calf muscles.

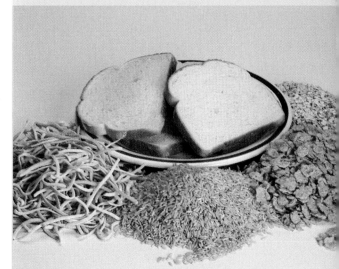

What Do the Parts of the Nervous System Do?

Your **nervous** (NUHR·vuhs) **system** is made up of organs that control all your body actions. Certain cells in these organs receive and send messages to all body parts. These messages tell your body what to do.

Your brain Your *brain* is an organ that receives and sends messages to all your body parts. Your brain gets information from your senses. Your five senses are hearing, seeing, touching, tasting, and smelling. The sense organs—ears, eyes, skin, tongue, and nose—send messages to your brain. Suppose you want to catch a ball. Messages from your brain tell your eyes to follow the ball. Your brain sends messages that signal the muscles in your hands to catch the ball.

Your nerves *Nerves* are groups of special cells in your body that carry messages from your sense organs to your brain. Suppose a record is playing. Nerve cells in your ear send the message to the hearing center in your brain. You hear the music. If you touch something hot, nerve cells in your skin send a message to your brain. Your brain sends a message to your muscles to pull your hand away.

Your spinal cord Your *spinal cord* is a long column of nerve cells that attaches to your brain. Your spinal cord allows messages to travel between your brain and other parts of your body. Your spinal cord is surrounded by your spine. Your vertebrae make up your spine.

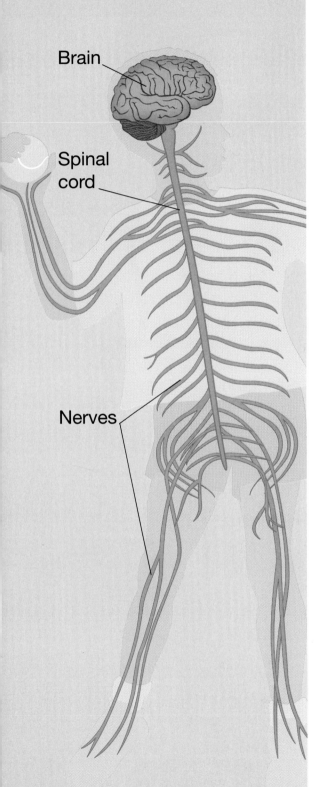

Brain

Spinal cord

Nerves

Wearing a safety belt protects your brain and spinal cord if you are in a car accident. Perhaps you have seen a person who cannot move his or her body from the waist down. This person might have a spinal cord injury.

Being drug-free helps protect nerve cells. Alcohol is a depressant drug. It slows down the action of nerve cells. Marijuana is a harmful drug. It changes body senses. Alcohol and marijuana (MEHR·uh·WAH·nuh) harm nerve cells.

Wearing a mask keeps you from breathing fumes that harm nerve cells. Fumes from cleaners, paints, and glues can harm nerve cells. You can wear a mask to keep from breathing the fumes. A mask can be bought at a hardware store or paint store.

Keeping a window open keeps you from breathing fumes that harm nerve cells. Suppose you do projects with paste or glue. Suppose you paint or your parents paint. Suppose you use household cleaners to scrub the tub. You can keep a window open to lessen the fumes.

Wearing a helmet for physical activities protects your brain from injury. You need to wear a helmet if you bike or skate. You need to wear a helmet when you are the batter in a baseball game. Suppose you play football or ice hockey when you are older. You need a helmet for these sports, too.

What Do the Parts of the Digestive System Do?

The **digestive** (dy·JES·tiv) **system** is made up of organs that help your body use food. *Digestion* (dy·JES·chuhn) is a process of changing food you eat so it can be used by your body.

Your salivary glands Your *salivary* (SA·luh·VEHR·ee) *glands* are organs that make saliva. *Saliva* (suh·LY·vuh) is a liquid in your mouth that softens food. This makes it easier for your teeth to grind food. It makes it easier to swallow food. The softened food moves down a tube to your stomach.

Your stomach Your *stomach* is an organ that releases special juices to break down food. Food is changed into a thick paste. Then it moves into your small intestine.

Your small intestine Your *small intestine* is an organ that breaks down most of the food you eat into substances your body cells can use. Your blood carries these substances to your body cells.

Your large intestine Some food is not digested. It cannot be used by the body. It is solid waste. The *large intestine* is the body organ through which solid waste passes. It also is called the colon. Muscles move solid waste through the large intestine and out of the body.

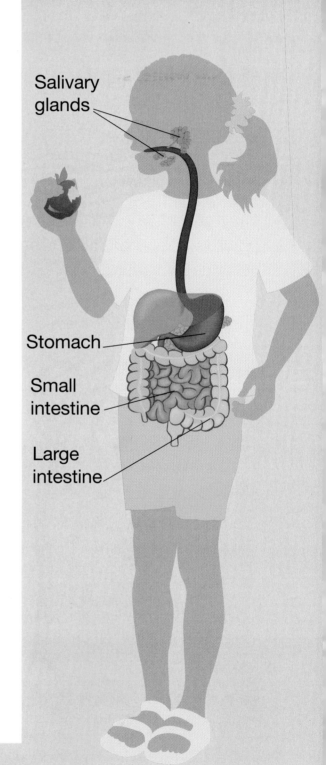

Salivary glands

Stomach

Small intestine

Large intestine

Chewing food helps digestion. When you eat slowly, you give saliva a chance to soften food. You chew longer and food is broken into smaller pieces. It is easier to swallow.

Eating fruits, vegetables, and fiber helps you have a daily bowel movement. A *bowel movement* is the movement of solid waste out of your body. This keeps the large intestine or colon clean. Fruits, vegetables, and grains have fiber in them. Fiber is the part of grains and plant foods that cannot be digested. Grains like whole wheat bread and bran cereals have fiber in them. Apples, oranges, broccoli, and celery have fiber in them.

Drinking water helps with digestion. Nearly two-thirds of your body is water. You should drink eight glasses of water a day. This helps you digest food more easily. Water also helps you have a daily bowel movement.

Physical activity helps you have a daily bowel movement. Regular physical activity helps muscles work as they should. Muscles help move solid wastes through the large intestine and out of the body.

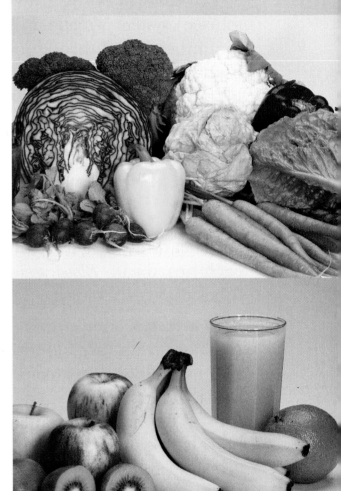

What Do the Parts of the Circulatory System Do?

The **circulatory** (SUHR·kyuh·luh·tohr·ee) **system** is made up of organs that move blood throughout your body. Your heart, blood, and blood vessels are part of your circulatory system.

Your heart Your *heart* is a muscular organ that pumps blood. Your heart muscle pumps blood into your blood vessels with each heartbeat. Your heart muscle gets rest between each heartbeat. *Blood vessels* are tubes that carry blood.

Your arteries Your *arteries* (AHR·tuh·reez) are blood vessels that take blood away from your heart. They carry oxygen to body cells. They carry substances that body cells use for energy. The arteries can change in size. They can be narrow. They can widen. Fatty foods that you eat can stick to the walls of your arteries.

Your veins Your *veins* are blood vessels that bring blood back to your heart. They have valves in them to keep blood from flowing backwards. Muscles in your legs push against veins. This helps blood go back up to the heart.

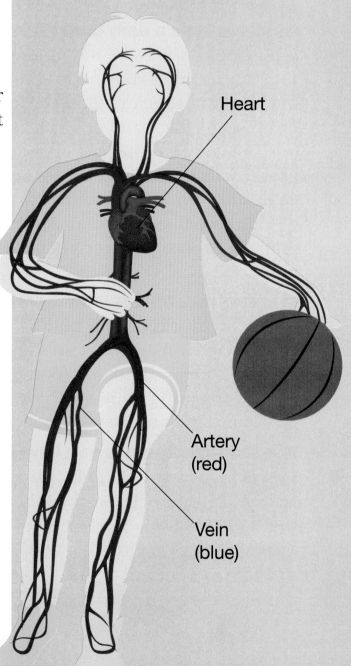

Heart

Artery (red)

Vein (blue)

Physical activity makes your heart muscle strong and keeps fat from sticking to arteries. Walking, running, dancing, swimming, and biking are good for your heart and arteries.

Low-fat foods are better for your arteries than high-fat foods. They are less likely to stick to artery walls. You can drink skim milk or 2 percent milk. You can eat low-fat cheese or low-fat ice cream.

Using tobacco is harmful to your heart and arteries. Tobacco products have nicotine in them. Suppose you try tobacco. Tobacco speeds up your heart. Your heart beats more often. Your arteries get narrow. Your blood pressure goes up.

Sensing Your World

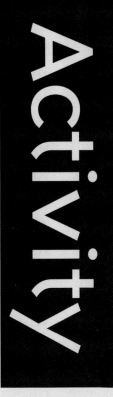

Life Skill

• **I will care for my body systems.**

Materials: Item in a sock to touch, safe substance to smell, tape of a sound, close-up picture of a common object, food item to taste, paper, pencil

Directions: Follow the directions below to learn how you use each sense to identify things.

1. **Your teacher will have you taste something.** Write down what you think you tasted.
2. **Your teacher will have you smell something.** Write down what you think you smelled.
3. **Your teacher will have you look at a picture.** Write down what you think the picture showed.
4. **Your teacher will have you listen to a sound.** Write down what you think you heard.
5. **Your teacher will have you touch an object.** Write down what you think you touched.
6. **Compare your answers with your classmates.** Did you all guess correctly?

What Do the Parts of the Respiratory System Do?

The **respiratory** (RES·puh·ruh·TOR·ee) **system** is made up of organs that help you use the air you breathe. You breathe in, or inhale, air through your mouth and nose.

Your nose Your *nose* is an organ that draws air into your body and allows you to smell things. There are nerve cells in your nose that help you smell.

Your throat Your *throat* is the passage between your mouth and your windpipe. It also is the passage between your mouth and the tube that goes to the stomach.

Your windpipe Your *windpipe* is a tube that goes from your throat to your lungs. Your windpipe must be kept clear so you can breathe.

Your lungs Your *lungs* are organs that put oxygen into the blood and take carbon dioxide out of the blood. *Oxygen* (AHK·si·juhn) is a gas needed for you to live. *Carbon dioxide* (KAR·buhn dy·AHK·SYD) is a gas that is a waste product from your cells. When you breathe in, air goes into your lungs. Your blood picks up oxygen and takes it to body cells. Your blood picks up carbon dioxide from body cells. It returns it to the lungs. When you breathe out, carbon dioxide leaves your body.

What Do Cilia Do?

Cilia are tiny hairs that line the air passages. They beat back and forth to keep particles from getting in your lungs. Smoke from cigars and cigarettes makes cilia not work.

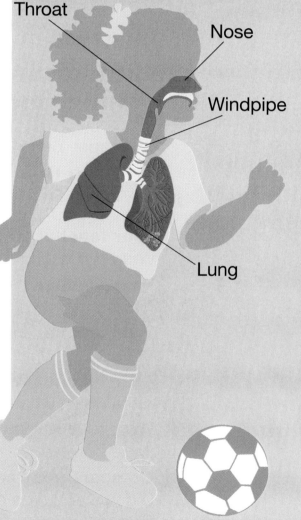

Throat

Nose

Windpipe

Lung

Physical activity makes muscles that help lungs work get strong. Then you can breathe in more air. You can exhale more air. Walking, running, swimming, and biking make these muscles strong.

Being smoke-free keeps you from having diseases of the respiratory system. You will get fewer colds. You will not get other conditions that harm the windpipe. You will lessen the chance that you will ever have lung cancer.

Having good posture helps your lungs work as they should. If you slouch over, your lungs do not have the space they need to work well.

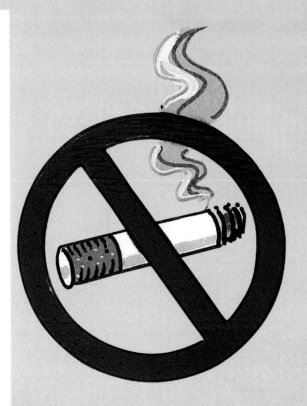

Lesson 10

Review

Vocabulary

Write a separate sentence using each vocabulary word listed on page 67.

Health Content

1. What do the parts of the skeletal system do? **page 68**

2. What do the parts of the muscular system do? **page 70**

3. What do the parts of the nervous system do? **page 72**

4. What do the parts of the digestive system do? **page 74** What do the parts of the circulatory system do? **page 76**

5. What do the parts of the respiratory system do? **page 78**

Growing and Changing

Vocabulary

puberty: the stage in life when a person's body changes to become an adult.

hearing aid: a small device that makes sounds louder.

arthritis: a condition in which joints become swollen and sore.

stroke: a condition that is caused by a blocked or broken blood vessel in the brain.

Life Skills

- I will accept how my body changes as I grow.
- I will learn the stages of the life cycle.
- I will choose habits for healthful growth and aging.

You are growing and changing right now. Your body is growing. You are doing new things. You are making new friends. As you get older, your body will keep changing. You can practice habits to stay healthy throughout your life.

The Lesson Objectives

- List signs you are growing.
- Explain how older adults change.

What Are Signs I Am Growing?

You might outgrow your clothes quickly. You might need new shoes often. You are growing in many ways.

Your body grows as you get older. You grow about two inches taller each year. You gain about six or seven pounds each year. This growth happens in spurts, or a certain amount at a time. You might be taller or shorter than some of your classmates. This is because everyone grows at different speeds. Later, a classmate who was shorter than others might grow taller. You might have gaps in your mouth where you have lost baby teeth. You might have grown some of your permanent teeth.

Your mind grows as you get older. You are better able to learn new things. You can handle harder subjects in school. You can do more things by yourself. You do chores without being told. This means you are becoming more responsible. People will trust you to be more responsible. They know that you will try to do your best.

Your relationships grow as you get older. The activities you enjoy with friends and family might change. You keep spending time with old friends. You make new friends. You might enjoy different activities with some friends than with others. This is normal. You might have one or two best friends.

What Is Puberty?

You are moving toward puberty. **Puberty** (PYOO·ber·tee) is the stage in life when a person's body changes to become an adult. Girls usually begin puberty between ages 10 and 12. Boys usually reach puberty around age 12 or 13. During puberty, you will go through a big growth spurt. Other changes will occur that will help you become an adult.

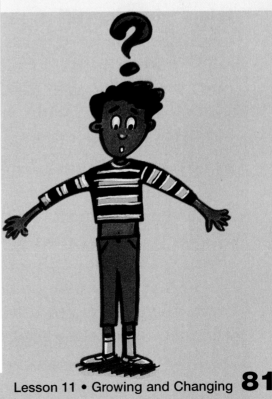

How Do Older Adults Change?

Just as you are going through many changes, adults change as they get older.

Eyesight might change As adults get older, their eyesight changes. They might need glasses or contacts, even if they did not need them when they were younger. They might need a special kind of glasses called bifocals. *Bifocals* (BY·FOH·kuhlz) are a kind of eyeglasses that allow a person to see nearby objects through one part and faraway objects through another part.

Hearing might change Some older adults have trouble hearing. They might ask you to repeat things you have said. They might want to have the TV or radio turned up louder. They might use hearing aids. A **hearing aid** is a small device that makes sounds louder.

Joints might be stiff Some older adults might seem to move more slowly. They might have arthritis. **Arthritis** (ar·THRY·tuhs) is a condition in which joints become swollen and sore. Arthritis can make it hard to walk or bend over.

Symptoms of disease might appear You might know an older adult who cannot speak clearly or move a body part. These problems can be caused by a stroke. A **stroke** is a condition that is caused by a blocked or broken blood vessel in the brain. Be patient and listen to a person who cannot speak clearly.

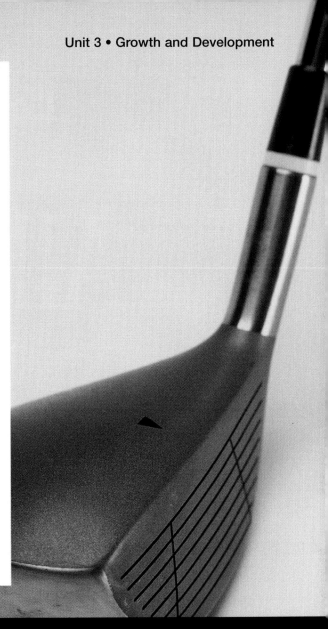

Ways to Be in Good Health When You Are Older

Begin now to eat healthful foods. You will learn more about healthful eating in Unit 4. Eat plenty of fruits, vegetables, and fiber. Limit the amount of fatty foods you eat.

Begin now to get plenty of physical activity. Walk, run, bike, skate, swim, or do other activities. Play sports you enjoy. Continue to get physical activity as you get older.

Begin now to work on hobbies you enjoy. A *hobby* is something you like to do in your spare time. A hobby helps you build skills. It gives you a way to ease stress. You can share hobbies with other people. You can make new friends. Having friends helps you stay in good health as you get older.

Lesson 11

Review

Vocabulary

Write a separate sentence using each vocabulary word listed on page 80.

Health Content

1. How is your body growing? **page 81**

2. How is your mind growing? **page 81**

3. How are your relationships growing? **page 81**

4. What are ways older adults might change? **page 82**

5. What are three habits you can form now to help you stay healthy as you get older? **pages 82–83**

All of Me

Vocabulary

heredity: the traits you get from your birth parents.

personality: the blend of ways you look, think, act, and feel.

self-esteem: the way you feel about yourself.

disability: something that changes a person's ability to do certain things.

hearing aid: a small device that makes sounds louder.

Life Skills

- I will be glad that I am unique.
- I will discover my learning style.

Everyone is special. You have many things about you that are special. Some people also have special needs. You can understand the special needs other people might have. You also can learn skills to study well. When you know how to study, you are less likely to feel stressed before a test. You know you can handle it.

The Lesson Objectives

- Explain what makes you special.
- Explain how you can have good study habits.
- Explain what you can do if you get stressed before a test.
- List special needs people might have.

What Makes Me Special?

Your heredity makes you special. Your **heredity** is the traits you get from your birth parents. Traits include hair color, eye color, skin color, face shape, and others. For example, you might have brown hair or blond hair or red hair or black hair. You probably look like your mother in some ways and like your father in other ways. No one has the exact group of traits that you have.

Your personality makes you special. Your **personality** is the blend of ways you look, think, act, and feel. The way you behave is part of your personality. The way you treat other people is part of your personality. You need to behave in responsible ways. You need to treat others with respect. You might be quiet, or you might like to talk. This is part of your personality.

The activities you enjoy make you special. You might like to read or write stories. You might like to play a sport or make crafts. When you do these activities, you become good at them. You might know more about them than other people do. You have something to do in your free time.

What Is Self-Esteem?

Self-esteem is the way you feel about yourself. Positive self-esteem is good feelings about yourself. You can have positive self-esteem. Choose responsible actions. Other people will feel good about you, too. They will respect you.

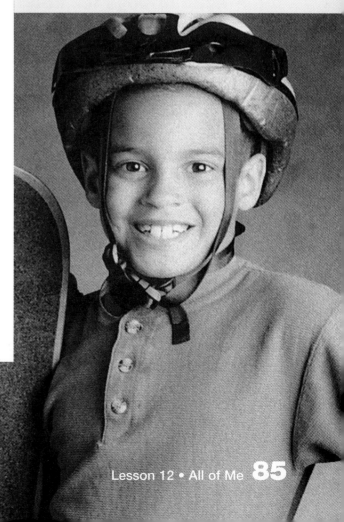

How Can I Have Good Study Habits?

To *study* is to review and practice the things you have learned. Here are some tips for good study habits.

- **Write down facts you want to remember.** Write down facts that will be on your test. Write down anything that will help you understand what you are learning. This is called taking notes.

- **Study at the same time every day, if you can.** Plan a specific time to study. Study in a quiet place that has good light. Make sure you have plenty of pencils and paper.

- **Read through the notes you took in class.** You might use a special marker to highlight facts.

- **Review information in your textbook.** Ask your parents or guardian to help you with anything you do not understand. Or make a note to ask your teacher.

- **Brainstorm ideas on scrap paper.** To brainstorm is to write down all the ideas you think of. Then you can look at you list and choose the best idea.

Ask for Help!

Do not be afraid to ask for help if you do not understand something you study. Many school subjects build on things you have already learned. If you do not understand something, it might be hard to learn the next facts in that subject.

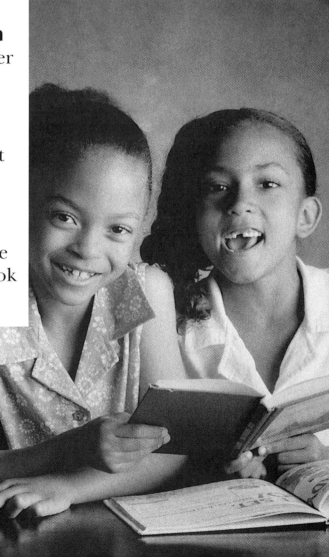

What Can I Do If I Get Stressed Before a Test?

You might feel stressed before you take a test. This is normal. A little stress helps you focus on the test. If you study well, you will not be too worried before a test.

Don't wait until the last minute to study for a test. You already will know most of the information if you study a little bit every day. You will have had time to get help with anything you do not understand. If you still need help, ask for it at least one day before the test.

Do something new with the facts you have learned to help you remember them. For example, you might draw pictures of things you want to remember. You might make a chart that shows the facts you have learned. You might make flash cards to help you remember facts. You might make up a song using the facts you have learned. You might write a story using the facts.

Get a good night's sleep before the test.

Eat a healthful breakfast.

Be ready to take the test. Make sure you have all the supplies you will need. Sharpen your pencils. Get out some scrap paper if you are allowed to use it.

Close your eyes and take a few slow, deep breaths through your nose. Let them out slowly. Then open your eyes, smile, and picture a big "A+" at the top of your test!

Make a Deck of Flash Cards

Write a question on the front of each card. Write the answer to the question on the back of the card. Ask your parent, guardian, sister, or brother to show you the question sides of the flash cards. You must give the correct answer to each question.

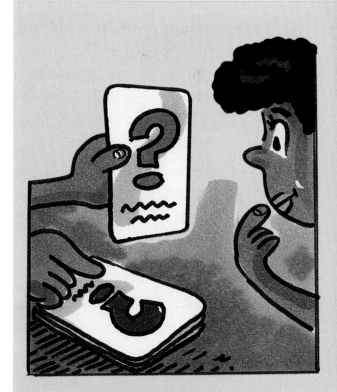

What Are Special Needs People Might Have?

You might know someone who has a special need. He or she might have a disability. A **disability** (DI·suh·BI·luh·tee) is something that changes a person's ability to do certain things.

Seeing Some people cannot see. Or they might be able to see only certain things. These people might use a cane to help them move around. They might have a dog that helps them. A person who is blind might have books in Braille. *Braille* is a way of writing with raised dots that blind people can touch to read.

Hearing and speaking Some people cannot hear well. They might use a hearing aid. A **hearing aid** is a small device that makes sounds louder. It is worn in the ear. A person who cannot hear might use sign language. *Sign language* is a way to communicate by using the hands and arms instead of speaking.

Moving Some people need to use a wheelchair. People who use wheelchairs might have been injured or have a certain disease.

Learning A *learning disability* is something that causes a person to have trouble learning. People who have learning disabilities might take special classes. They might have a tutor who helps them with their schoolwork.

Help a Friend Who Has a Disability

- Treat a person who has a disability the same way you would treat anyone else.

- Talk directly to the person, even if he or she cannot hear.

- Tell your name to a person who cannot see. Tell him or her the names of anyone with you. Say the name of the person to whom you are speaking.

- Ask permission before you help a person who has a disability. Listen to any directions he or she gives you about how to help.

- Do not pet a helper dog while it is helping a person who has a disability. The dog is working. If the dog is resting, ask permission before you pet it.

Homework Calendar

Activity

Life Skill

● **I will develop my learning style.**

Materials: Paper, pencil, colored markers

Directions: Follow the directions below to make a calendar to help you study.

1. **Draw a calendar for the next two weeks.** Make a space for each day. Make each space big enough to write several things in it.

2. **Write any tests that you know you will have on your calendar.** Write each homework assignment your teacher gives you on your calendar. Cross off each assignment when you finish it.

3. **Make a new one when the two weeks have passed.**

Lesson 12

Review

Vocabulary

Write a separate sentence using each vocabulary word listed on page 84.

Health Content

1. What makes you special? **page 85**
2. How can you have good study habits? **page 86**
3. What can you do if you get stressed before a test? **page 87**
4. What are special needs people might have? **page 88**
5. How can you help a friend who has a disability? **page 88**

Unit 3 Review

Health Content

1. What are exercises that make bones strong? **Lesson 10 page 69**

2. What are foods that keep muscles healthy? **Lesson 10 page 71**

3. How can you protect your nervous system? **Lesson 10 page 73**

4. What do the parts of the circulatory system do? **Lesson 10 page 76**

5. What are ways your mind is growing? **Lesson 11 page 81**

6. What are ways you can stay healthy as you get older? **Lesson 11 pages 82–83**

7. How might older adults change? **Lesson 11 pages 82–83**

8. What are good study habits you can have? **Lesson 12 page 86**

9. How can you deal with stress before a test? **Lesson 12 page 87**

10. What are ways you can help a friend who has a disability? **Lesson 12 page 88**

Guidelines for Making Responsible Decisions™

Your friend calls and asks you to come over. But it is the time of day when you usually study. Answer "yes" or "no" to each of the following questions. Explain each answer.

1. Is it healthful to go to your friend's house when you usually study?

2. Is it safe to go to your friend's house when you usually study?

3. Do you follow rules and laws if you go to your friend's house when you usually study?

4. Do you show respect for yourself and others if you go to your friend's house when you usually study?

5. Do you follow your family's guidelines if you go to your friend's house when you usually study?

6. Do you show good character if you go to your friend's house when you usually study?

What is the responsible decision to make?

Vocabulary

Number a sheet of paper from 1–10. Read each definition. Next to each number on your sheet of paper, write the vocabulary word that matches the definition.

body system	arthritis
nervous system	heredity
digestive system	personality
puberty	self-esteem
hobby	disability

1. Something that changes a person's ability to do certain things. **Lesson 12**

2. The stage in life when a person's body changes to become an adult. **Lesson 11**

3. The blend of ways you look, think, act, and feel. **Lesson 12**

4. Organs that help your body use food. **Lesson 10**

5. A condition in which joints become swollen and sore. **Lesson 11**

6. A group of organs that work together to do a certain job. **Lesson 10**

7. The way you feel about yourself. **Lesson 12**

8. Something you like to do in your spare time. **Lesson 11**

9. The traits you get from your birth parents. **Lesson 12**

10. Organs that control all your body actions. **Lesson 10**

Health Literacy

Effective Communication

Draw a picture of one of the body systems described in Lesson 10. Label the parts of the body system. Hang the picture in your classroom.

Self-Directed Learning

Make a crossword puzzle using the names of the organs described in Lesson 10. Include at least ten organs. Remember to write clues for your puzzle.

Critical Thinking

Why do you need to form habits now that will help you stay healthy when you are an older adult? Answer the question on a separate sheet of paper.

Responsible Citizenship

Make a poster that shows ways to have good study habits. Hang the poster in your classroom.

Family Involvement

Talk to your parents or guardian about ways you can help older adults you know. Plan to spend time with an older adult.

Unit 4

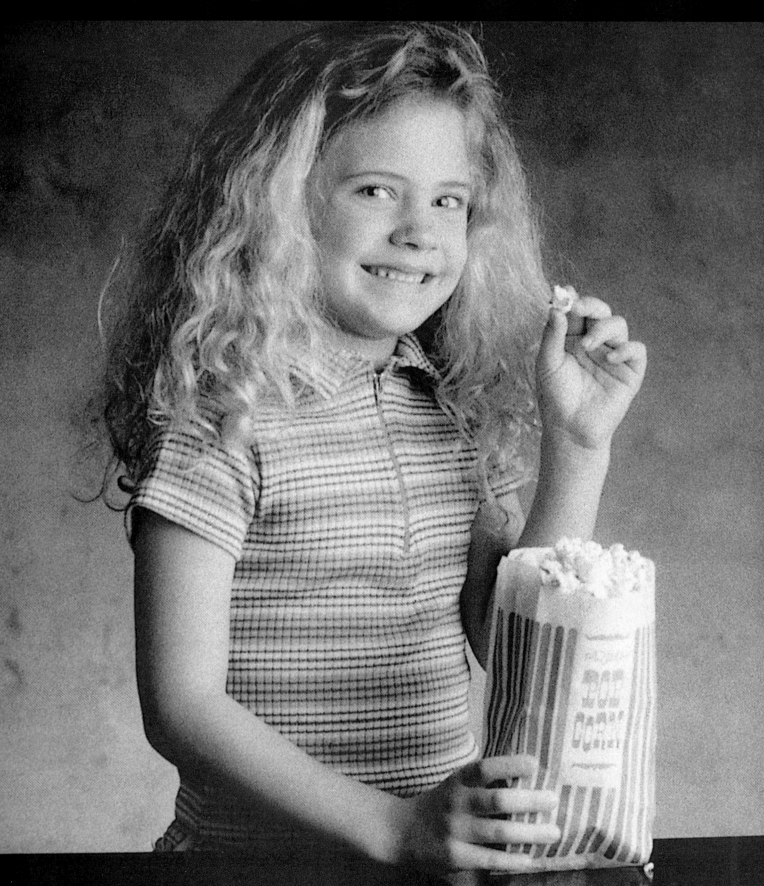

Nutrition

Nutrition in Action

Vocabulary

nutrient: a material in food that is used by the body.

energy: the ability to do work.

carbohydrates: nutrients that supply the main source of energy for your body.

vitamins: nutrients that help your body use proteins, carbohydrates, and fats.

Food Guide Pyramid: a guide that tells how many servings are needed from each food group each day.

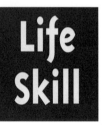

Life Skill

● **I will eat the correct number of servings from the Food Guide Pyramid.**

You can plan meals to include all the foods you need each day. You can be healthy and strong when you eat a healthful diet. A **nutrient** (NOO·tree·uhnt) is a material in food that is used by the body. Some nutrients help you grow. Some provide energy for you to run and play. **Energy** is the ability to do work.

The Lesson Objectives

● Explain how your body uses nutrients.

● Discuss how you can get all the nutrients you need.

How Does My Body Use Nutrients?

Carbohydrates (kahr·boh·HY·draytes) are nutrients that supply the main source of energy for your body. *Sugars* are carbohydrates that provide quick energy. Some sugars are found in fruits and other food. *Starches* are carbohydrates that provide energy that lasts a long time. Starches are found in bread, pasta, potatoes, and beans.

Proteins (PROH·teenz) are nutrients that are used to grow and repair body cells. Proteins are found in meat, fish, eggs, milk, yogurt, cheese, and beans.

Fats are nutrients that are used for energy and to keep the body warm. Fats help the cells get and use vitamins. Fats are found in meat, dairy products, oil, and margarine.

Vitamins (VY·tuh·muhnz) are nutrients that help your body use proteins, carbohydrates, and fats. Eat plenty of vegetables and other healthful foods to get all the vitamins you need.

Minerals are nutrients that are used to help your body work as it should. Some minerals you need are calcium, phosphorus, and iron. You can get the minerals you need by eating a healthful diet.

Water is a nutrient that is used for body processes. Water is used for digestion. Water makes up part of blood. You get water by drinking it. You get it from fruits and vegetables, too.

Eat Your Fiber

Fiber is the part of grains and plant foods that cannot be digested. You need fiber to help you have a daily bowel movement. Fiber also can protect you from some diseases, such as cancer. Eat whole-grain cereals, breads, and fruits and vegetables to get plenty of fiber.

Drink Little Soda Pop

You might think drinking soda pop will give you the water you need. But soda pop has substances that make you urinate more. Your body cannot use the water from the soda pop. Drink water or juice instead of soda pop.

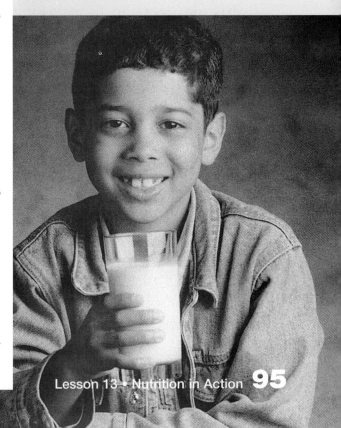

How Can I Get All the Nutrients I Need?

You can get all the nutrients you need from a healthful diet. The U.S. Department of Agriculture has made a guide to help you plan healthful meals. This guide is called the Food Guide Pyramid. The **Food Guide Pyramid** is a guide that tells how many servings are needed from each food group each day.

Look at the Food Guide Pyramid. You will see that the biggest part, the bottom of the pyramid, is the Bread, Cereal, Rice, and Pasta Group. You should eat more servings from this group than from any other group. Foods from this food group give you vitamins, minerals, carbohydrates, and fiber. You need to eat 6 to 11 servings from this group each day. A serving is:

1 slice of bread or

1/2 of a bagel or English muffin or

1 ounce of ready-to-eat cereal or

1/2 cup of cooked cereal, rice, or pasta or

5 to 6 small crackers

The next group up the pyramid is the Vegetable Group. Foods from this group give you vitamins, minerals, and fiber. You need to eat 3 to 5 servings from this group each day. A serving is:

1 cup raw, leafy vegetables or

1/2 cup cooked or chopped raw vegetables or

3/4 cup vegetable juice

Beside the Vegetable Group is the Fruit Group. Fruits give you vitamins, minerals, and carbohydrates, including fiber. You need to eat 2 to 4 servings from this group each day. A serving is:

1 medium apple, banana, orange, or pear or

1/2 cup chopped, cooked, canned, or mixed fruit or

3/4 cup fruit juice

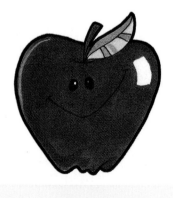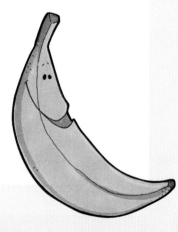

Farther up the pyramid, you will see the Milk, Yogurt, and Cheese Group. These foods give you calcium and protein. Choose low-fat products, such as skim milk and fat-free yogurt. You need to eat 2 to 3 servings from this group each day. A serving is:

1 cup milk or yogurt or

1-1/2 ounces of natural cheese or

2 ounces of processed cheese

Next is the Meat, Poultry, Fish, Dry Beans, Eggs, and Nuts Group. These foods give you protein, vitamins, and minerals. Meats, poultry, fish, and eggs can be high in fat. Eat lean meats, beans, and egg whites to cut down on fat. You need to eat 2 to 3 servings from this group each day. A serving is:

2 to 3 ounces of cooked lean meat, poultry, or fish or

1/2 cup cooked beans or

1 egg or

2 tablespoons of peanut butter or

1/3 cup nuts

The tiny top of the pyramid includes Fats, Oils, and Sweets. You do not need to eat any of these foods to be healthy. These foods are high in fat and sugar. They have few vitamins and minerals. Foods in this group are cakes, candies, cookies, butter, margarine, salad dressing, soda pop, and other "junk foods."

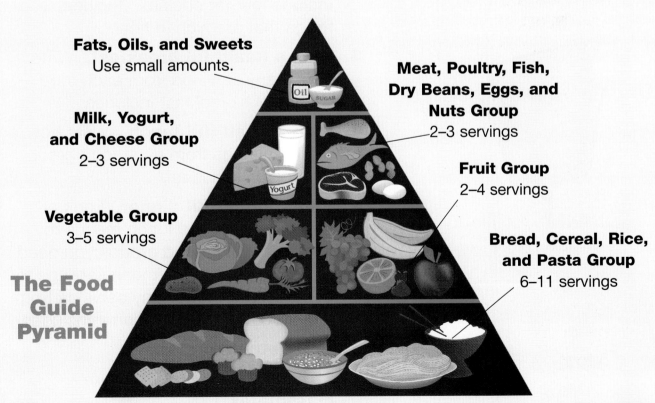

Fats, Oils, and Sweets
Use small amounts.

Milk, Yogurt,
and Cheese Group
2–3 servings

Meat, Poultry, Fish,
Dry Beans, Eggs, and
Nuts Group
2–3 servings

Vegetable Group
3–5 servings

Fruit Group
2–4 servings

Bread, Cereal, Rice,
and Pasta Group
6–11 servings

The Food
Guide
Pyramid

Plan a Healthful Menu

Activity

Life Skill

• I will eat the correct number of servings from the Food Guide Pyramid.

Materials: Paper, pencil, markers

Directions: Suppose you own a restaurant. Follow the directions below to plan healthful meals.

1. **Think of a name for your restaurant.** Write the name at the top of your sheet of paper. Write "Menu" under the name.

2. **Suppose a person will eat all three meals at your restaurant on one day.** Write a menu that will include the right number of servings for the day from each food group. Include low-fat choices. Include foods that are high in fiber.

3. **Plan a healthful breakfast.** Write how many servings from each food group your breakfast includes.

4. **Plan a healthful lunch.** Write how many servings from each food group your lunch includes.

5. **Plan a healthful dinner.** Look at your breakfast and lunch menus to see from which food groups you need more servings. Plan those servings for dinner. Write how many servings from each food group your dinner includes.

6. **Decorate your menu.**

7. **Share your menu with your classmates.**

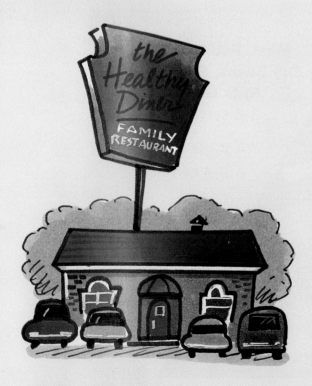

Use... Guidelines for Making Responsible Decisions™

Situation:

You drink a lot of soda pop. You do not like to drink water.

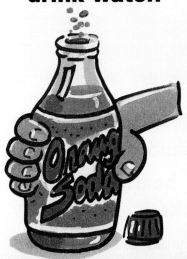

Response:

Answer "yes" or "no" to each of the following questions. Explain each answer.

1. Is it healthful to drink soda pop instead of water?

2. Is it safe to drink soda pop instead of water?

3. Do you follow rules and laws if you drink soda pop instead of water?

4. Do you show respect for yourself and others if you drink soda pop instead of water?

5. Do you follow your family's guidelines if you drink soda pop instead of water?

6. Do you show good character if you drink soda pop instead of water?

What is the responsible decision to make?

Lesson 13

Review

Vocabulary

Write a separate sentence using each vocabulary word listed on page 94.

Health Content

1. What are six nutrients your body needs? **page 95**

2. How does your body use each of the six nutrients? **page 95**

3. How can you get all the nutrients you need? **pages 96–97**

4. What is a serving from the Bread, Cereal, Rice, and Pasta Group? **pages 96–97**

5. What is a serving from the Milk, Yogurt, and Cheese Group? **pages 96–97**

Going for the Dietary Guidelines

Vocabulary

Dietary Guidelines: suggested goals for eating to help you stay healthy and live longer.

fiber: the part of grains and plant foods that cannot be digested.

natural sugar: the sugar that is in foods and has not been added.

alcohol: a drug found in some beverages that slows down the body.

Life Skills

- I will follow the Dietary Guidelines.
- I will eat healthful meals and snacks.
- I will stay at a healthful weight.

The **Dietary Guidelines** are suggested goals for eating to help you stay healthy and live longer. There are seven Dietary Guidelines. Follow these seven Dietary Guidelines to help you make healthful food choices.

The Lesson Objectives

- Explain how you can follow the seven Dietary Guidelines.

How Can I Follow the Dietary Guidelines?

Dietary Guideline 1: Eat a variety of foods.

Each food belongs to one of the groups on the Food Guide Pyramid. Always eat the right number of servings from each food group on the Food Guide Pyramid. Eat different foods from each food group every day. For example, you need to eat at least three servings from the Vegetable Group each day. Suppose you eat three servings of carrots. Carrots have vitamin A in them. They do not have some of the other vitamins you can get from vegetables. Suppose you eat a serving of carrots, a serving of broccoli, and a potato. You will get a better variety of vitamins and minerals.

Dietary Guideline 2: Balance the food you eat with physical activity—stay at a healthful weight.

Your body works best when you are at the weight that is right for you. Your doctor can tell you how much you should weigh. You might weigh too much or too little for your height and build. Or you might be at a healthful weight.

To stay at a healthful weight, get plenty of physical activity. Choose healthful foods. You can choose to eat few foods that are high in fat and sugar. You can eat plenty of fruits, vegetables, and fiber.

Do Not Skip Breakfast

Do you eat breakfast? You should. Eating breakfast gives you energy to start your day right. Include some protein, fiber, and fruits or vegetables in your breakfast. Try fruit on whole-grain cereal with skim milk. Scramble some egg whites with salsa and vegetables, and toast some whole-grain bread as a side dish. Whip up some oatmeal with raisins, and eat a cup of yogurt to top it off.

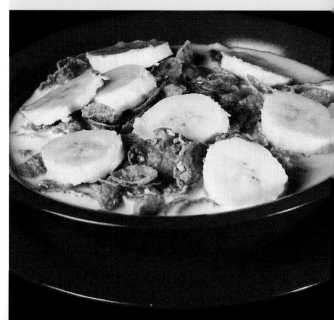

Dietary Guideline 3: Eat few fatty foods.

Suppose you eat lots of fatty foods. Fats can stick to your artery walls. Then it is harder for blood to flow through arteries. Your heart has to work very hard.

Some foods with fat are better for your health than others. Fats that stick to your artery walls are in foods that come from animals. Some examples are meat, milk, butter, ice cream, and cheese. Some fats that stick to your artery walls come from vegetable fat.

Limit the amount of foods you eat from animals. Eat low-fat foods when you can. Drink skim milk. Eat low-fat ice cream and yogurt.

Dietary Guideline 4: Eat plenty of grains, vegetables, and fruits.

Grains, vegetables, and fruits give you vitamins and minerals. They give you fiber. **Fiber** is the part of grains and plant foods that cannot be digested. The skins of many fruits contain fiber. Leafy vegetables, such as lettuce and cabbage, have some fiber. Whole-grain breads and cereals have fiber.

Eat plenty of fruits and vegetables. Eat the skins of apples and pears. Eat whole-wheat bread and whole-grain cereals. Drink plenty of water. Eating foods that have fiber and drinking water will help you have regular bowel movements. Regular bowel movements help keep your digestive system healthy.

Easy Ways to Add Fruits and Vegetables

- Put sliced bananas or berries on your cereal.
- Drink 100 percent fruit or vegetable juice instead of soda pop or fruit punch.
- Have a salad instead of French fries.
- Order vegetables on your pizza instead of meat.

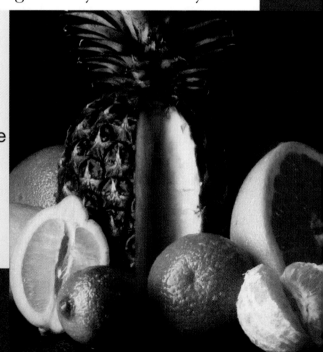

Dietary Guideline 5:
Eat small amounts of sugar.

Some foods, like apples and oranges, have natural sugar in them. Some vegetables also have natural sugar. **Natural sugar** is the sugar that is in foods and has not been added. Foods with natural sugar give you energy. They are healthful when you want to eat something sweet.

Sugar is added to many foods. Candy, cakes, and many soft drinks are made with added sugar. Sugar also is added to some cereals.

Your body needs some sugar. Get the sugar you need by eating fruits and vegetables. Cut down on foods to which sugar has been added. Too much sugar can cause cavities. Too much sugar can cause you to gain extra weight. For good health eat foods with natural sugars. Do not add sugar to fruits or cereals. Eat few foods made with added sugars.

Dietary Guideline 6:
Use little salt.

You need less than a teaspoon of salt each day. Too much salt might cause your heart to work too hard. Salt already is in many of the foods you eat. Salt is in many breads. It is in many canned foods, such as soups and vegetables. For good health add little or no salt to food. Do not add salt to water in which foods are cooked. Eat few salty snacks like potato chips and pretzels.

Dietary Guideline 7:
Do not drink alcohol.

Alcohol is a drug found in some beverages that slows down the body. Alcohol can make it hard for you to think. Alcohol can harm body organs. It is against the law for you to drink alcohol.

Beware of MSG

MSG is a substance used to flavor foods. It is very high in salt. Asian foods sometimes have MSG. Canned foods such as soup sometimes have MSG. Some people have side effects if they eat foods that have MSG. They might get a headache. They might have a hard time breathing. Read the label or the menu. Try to avoid foods that have MSG.

Health Behavior Contract

Copy the health behavior contract on a separate sheet of paper.

DO NOT WRITE IN THIS BOOK.

Name:_____ **Date:**_____

Life Skill: I will follow the Dietary Guidelines.

Effect on My Health: I get the nutrients I need when I follow the Dietary Guidelines. I eat a variety of foods. I stay at a healthful weight. I eat few fatty foods. I eat foods that are low in sugar and salt. I eat plenty of fiber. I lower my risk of having fat stick to my artery walls. I lower my risk of cancer and heart disease. I do not drink alcohol.

My Plan: I will follow the Dietary Guidelines by choosing healthful foods. I will write down everything I eat for one week. At the end of each day, I will look at what I have eaten. I will see whether I followed each Dietary Guideline. Suppose I eat a food that does not follow the Dietary Guidelines. I will write the name of a food I could choose instead. I will make a mark on my calendar each day that I follow the Dietary Guidelines.

	M	T	W	Th	F	S	S

How My Plan Worked: (Complete after one week.)

Guideline Reminder

Life Skill

- I will follow the Dietary Guidelines.

Materials: Construction paper, scissors, markers

Directions: Follow the directions below to make a "Guideline Reminder" to help you remember the Dietary Guidelines.

Activity

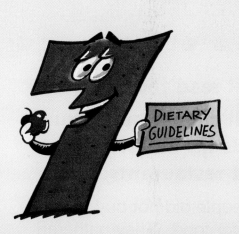

DIETARY GUIDELINES

1. **Draw the outline of a large "7" on the construction paper.** Cut out the shape. The shape will be your Guideline Reminder.

2. **Write one of the seven Dietary Guidelines on your Guideline Reminder.**

3. **Decorate your Guideline Reminder.** Hang your Guideline Reminder in your kitchen.

Lesson 14

Review

Vocabulary

Write a separate sentence using each vocabulary word listed on page 100.

Health Content

1. How can you eat a variety of foods? **page 101**

2. How can you stay at a healthful weight? **page 101**

3. Why do you need to eat few fatty foods? **page 102**

4. Why do you need to eat foods with fiber every day? **page 102**

5. What are three ways you can use less sugar? **page 103**

Hunt for Healthful Foods

Vocabulary

advertisement: a paid announcement.

commercial: an ad on radio or television.

food label: a part of a package that lists the ingredients and nutrition information of a food.

fast food restaurant: a place that serves food quickly.

snack: food eaten between meals.

Life Skills

- I will read food labels.
- I will choose healthful foods if I eat at fast food restaurants.

Many years ago, people did not buy foods. They hunted animals for food. They gathered berries and other plants that grew wild. You and your family go to the grocery store. You go to a fast food restaurant and choose what you want. But there is something you have in common. You still must hunt for healthful foods.

The Lesson Objectives

- Explain what food companies do to get you to buy a food.
- List tips for grocery shopping with your parents or guardian.
- List tips for ordering foods at fast food restaurants.
- Explain how you can use the Dietary Guidelines to choose healthful snacks.

How Do Food Companies Try to Get Me to Buy a Food?

Everyone eats. Most people buy the food they eat. Many companies sell food. Each company wants you to buy the food it sells.

Food companies make foods that look or taste good. The companies know that children like foods that are sweet. Children like foods that have bright colors. Companies make food taste good so you will want it. They put sugar in cereals. They make cereal in fun shapes. They make foods that are fun to eat. You might be able to unroll a food. You might be able to dip a food in something.

Restaurants also offer special foods for children. They might have a "kids' meal." They might give a toy with the meal.

Food companies put foods in special packages. A package might be shaped like an animal. A package might have bright colors. A package might show cartoon characters.

Food companies pay lots of money for ads you will like. An **advertisement,** or ad, is a paid announcement. Ads might be printed in magazines or on posters. A **commercial** is an ad on radio or television. Food ads and commercials show children having fun while eating a food. They might include bright colors, flashing lights, and popular music. They show food that looks tasty and fun to eat.

What Are Tips for Grocery Shopping with My Parents or Guardian?

Suppose you shop for groceries with your parents or guardian. They might have a list of groceries they want to buy. You might make suggestions. While you shop, you might ask them to buy foods that are not on the list. You can follow tips to help you buy healthful foods.

Check food labels for information. Most foods have labels on them. A **food label** is a part of a package that lists the ingredients and nutrition information of a food. For example, a box of cereal might have a label that lists sugar, wheat, and salt. The ingredient that appears first makes up the largest part of the food.

Begin checking food labels. Suppose you learn that sugar is added to your cereal. Check the food label of another box of cereal. It has no added sugar. You might decide to buy the cereal without sugar.

Compare the prices for different brands. As a wise shopper, you compare the prices of foods. Suppose you see two brands of canned fruit. One brand costs less than the other. You check the food labels. Both have the same ingredients. You can buy the brand that costs less.

Nutrition Facts

Serving Size 9 Crackers (31g)
Serving Per Container about 13

Amount Per Serving

Calories 120   Calories from fat 15

	% Daily Value*
Total Fat 1.5g	**2**%
Saturated Fat 0.5g	**3**%
Cholesterol 0mg	**0**%
Sodium 210mg	**9**%
Total Carbohydrate 25g	**8**%
Dietary Fiber 1g	**4**%
Sugars 0g	
Protein 2g	

Vitamin A	0%	•	Vitamin C	0%
Calcium	0%	•	Iron	6%

* Percent Daily Values are based on a 2,000 calorie diet. Your daily values may be higher or lower depending on your calorie needs.

		Calories 2,000	2,500
Total Fat	Less than	65g	80g
Sat Fat	Less than	20g	25g
Cholesterol	Less than	300mg	300mg
Sodium	Less than	2,400mg	2,400mg
Total Carbohydrate		300g	375g
Dietary Fiber		25g	30g

A food label gives nutrition information and lists the ingredients of a food.

What Are Tips for Ordering Foods at Fast Food Restaurants?

A **fast food restaurant** is a place that serves food quickly. Fast food can be very tasty. But many food choices at fast food restaurants are high in fat. Here are some tips to help you order healthful foods at a fast food restaurant.

1. **Ask for nutrition information.** Many fast food restaurants have pamphlets that tell about their food. The pamphlets give much of the same information that would be on a food label. For example, they tell how many grams of fat are in the food.

2. **Order foods that help you get the right number of servings from the Food Guide Pyramid.** For example, you might choose a chicken sandwich on a whole-wheat bun. You might add tomatoes and lettuce to the sandwich. You might drink milk. This meal would give you two servings of grains, one to two servings of meat, a serving of vegetables, and a serving of milk.

3. **Order foods that help you follow the Dietary Guidelines.** The box at right shows how you can follow two of the Dietary Guidelines when you eat at a fast food restaurant.

Eat few fatty foods.
- Order a small or junior burger instead of a large burger.
- Skip the mayonnaise and special sauces.
- Order grilled chicken instead of fried chicken nuggets.
- Have a plain baked potato instead of French fries.
- Use low-fat dressing on your salad.
- Order pizza with vegetables instead of meat. Try your pizza without cheese.

Eat plenty of grains, vegetables, and fruits.
- Add lettuce and tomato to sandwiches.
- Order a side salad with vegetables, not meat or cheese.
- Order whole-wheat buns and pizza crust.

How Can I Use the Dietary Guidelines to Choose Healthful Snacks?

A **snack** is food eaten between meals. Many of the fun, colorful snacks sold in stores are high in sugar, fat, or both. These are not healthful snacks. They give you few vitamins or minerals. Follow the Dietary Guidelines to choose healthful snacks.

1. **Eat snacks that have a variety of nutrients.** You get more vitamins and minerals when you eat different foods for snacks. You get the servings you need from the Food Guide Pyramid.

2. **Eat snacks that help you stay at a healthful weight.** Eat low-calorie snacks. Do not eat junk foods. Choose fruit, vegetables, and low-fat products.

3. **Eat few fatty snacks.** Limit the amount of cake, candy bars, French fries, and burgers you eat. Choose low-fat yogurt and ice cream.

4. **Eat grains, vegetables, and fruits for snacks.** Eat whole-wheat crackers and bagels. Eat apples, bananas, oranges, berries, and kiwis. Try starfruit, mangoes, prunes, dates, and apricots. Eat carrot and celery sticks, radishes, and green pepper strips.

5. **Eat few snacks with sugar.** Eat foods with natural sugars. Do not add sugar to fruits or cereals. Eat few foods with added sugars.

6. **Eat few salty snacks.** Do not add salt to popcorn or fries. Eat unsalted chips, crackers, pretzels, and peanuts.

7. **Do not drink alcohol.**

Snacks to Try
- Frozen grapes or bananas
- Flavored rice cakes
- Low-fat yogurt and fruit
- Pretzels
- Graham crackers
- Air-popped popcorn (no butter)

Sing About Food Labels

Life Skill

• I will read food labels.

Materials: Paper, pencil

Directions: Follow the directions below to write a song verse about healthful eating.

1. **Sing the following song with your classmates.** Sing to the tune of "If You're Happy and You Know It, Clap Your Hands."

   If you want your blood to flow, watch your diet!

   If you want blood pressure low, watch your diet!

   If you want your heart to beat, then you watch what you eat.

   If you want the fat to go, watch your diet.

2. **Write another verse to this song.** Your verse should be about choosing healthful foods and reading food labels.

3. **Sing your song verse for your classmates.**

Activity

Lesson 15

Review

Vocabulary

Write a separate sentence using each vocabulary word listed on page 106.

Health Content

1. What are three things food companies do to try to get you to buy a food? **page 107**

2. What are tips for grocery shopping with your parents or guardian? **page 108**

3. What are three tips for ordering foods at fast food restaurants? **page 109**

4. How can you use two Dietary Guidelines to order foods at fast food restaurants? **page 109**

5. How can you use the Dietary Guidelines to choose healthful snacks? **page 110**

Please Pass the Table Manners

Vocabulary

table manners: polite ways to eat.

silverware: knives, forks, and spoons.

poultry: meat from chickens, turkeys, or other birds.

Life Skills

- I will use table manners.
- I will protect myself and others from germs in foods and beverages.

Suppose you are going to play soccer. You learn rules. When you follow the rules, you and others enjoy the game. You keep yourself and others from being injured. Suppose you are going to eat with others. There are rules for eating. They are called table manners. When you use table manners, you and others enjoy eating together. You keep food from being spilled. You do not spread germs.

The Lesson Objectives

- Discuss table manners you need to follow.
- Explain how you can keep your food safe.

What Table Manners Do I Need to Follow?

Table manners are polite ways to eat. You show respect for others when you have good table manners.

Place your napkin in your lap. Spread the napkin over your knees. Your napkin will protect your clothing in case you drop some food. You can wipe your hands on your napkin if you get food on them. You can wipe your mouth with your napkin.

Wait until everyone is served before you start eating. Someone might tell you to go ahead and eat before everyone has been served. Go ahead and eat if this happens.

Keep your silverware on your plate when you are not using it. Silverware is knives, forks, and spoons. Do not put a knife, fork, or spoon back on the table after you have used it. Food from the silverware might get on the table or tablecloth.

Chew with your mouth closed. No one wants to see the food in your mouth as you chew it. Chew your food carefully and swallow it before you open your mouth.

Take small bites. Do not gobble your food. Chew slowly.

Do not talk with your mouth full. Again, no one wants to see the food in your mouth. You are hard to understand when you talk with your mouth full. Wait to speak until you have swallowed your food.

Ask someone to pass you items you cannot reach. It is rude to reach across people or their plates to get foods. You can spill foods when you do this.

Say thanks to the person who made the food. You show good table manners when you thank a person for cooking a meal.

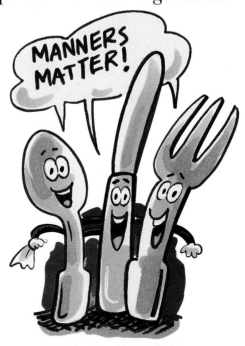

How Can I Keep Food Safe?

Sometimes, food contains germs. These germs can make you ill. Follow these rules to keep your food safe.

Wash your hands before you touch food. Wash your hands before you eat or prepare food.

Wash your hands after you touch raw meat or eggs. Raw meat and eggs can contain germs. Wash your hands to keep from spreading these germs.

Wash a cutting board that has been used to cut raw meat. Suppose you cut raw meat on a cutting board. Germs from the meat might get on the cutting board. Suppose you do not wash the cutting board. You cut carrots on the cutting board. The carrots might get germs on them from the meat. You might not cook the carrots. The germs on the carrots have not been killed. You eat them. The germs might make you ill.

Cook meat and poultry until they are done. **Poultry** is meat from chickens, turkeys, or other birds. Cooking kills the germs in meat and poultry.

Do not eat foods that contain raw eggs. Suppose you are baking cookies. You taste the cookie dough before it is baked. There are raw eggs in the cookie dough. Germs from raw eggs might make you sick.

Don't Share Germs!

Do not share silverware, drinking straws, or cups. Germs can be spread when people share eating utensils. Suppose you are eating ice cream. Your germs are on your spoon. You use your spoon to give your friend a taste of the ice cream. Your friend might get your germs. Then you might get your friend's germs when you take another bite.

Use... Guidelines for Making Responsible Decisions™

Situation:

You are eating dinner at a friend's house. You know you should thank your friend's mother for cooking. But you did not like the meal.

Response:

Answer "yes" or "no" to each of the following questions. Explain each answer.

1. Is it healthful to thank your friend's mother for cooking?

2. Is it safe to thank your friend's mother for cooking?

3. Do you follow rules and laws if you thank your friend's mother for cooking?

4. Do you show respect for yourself and others if you thank your friend's mother for cooking?

5. Do you follow your family's guidelines if you thank your friend's mother for cooking?

6. Do you show good character if you thank your friend's mother for cooking?

What is the responsible decision to make?

Lesson 16

Review

Vocabulary

Write a separate sentence using each vocabulary word listed on page 112.

Health Content

1. What are two reasons you should have good table manners? **page 113**

2. What are seven good table manners you need to follow? **page 113**

3. What are five ways you can keep food safe? **page 114**

4. Why should you wash a cutting board after you cut raw meat? **page 114**

5. Why should you not share silverware, straws, or cups? **page 114**

Unit 4 Review

Health Content

1. How does your body use each of the six nutrients it needs? **Lesson 13 page 95**

2. What are the five food groups on the Food Guide Pyramid? **Lesson 13 pages 96–97**

3. What counts as a serving from the Fruit Group? **Lesson 13 pages 96–97**

4. What are the seven Dietary Guidelines? **Lesson 14 pages 101–103**

5. How can you follow Dietary Guideline 2? **Lesson 14 page 101**

6. How do food companies try to get you to buy a food? **Lesson 15 page 107**

7. What are ways you can use the Dietary Guidelines to order foods at fast food restaurants? **Lesson 15 page 109**

8. What are ways you can use the Dietary Guidelines to choose healthful snacks? **Lesson 15 page 110**

9. Why do you need to have good table manners? **Lesson 16 page 113**

10. How can you keep food safe? **Lesson 16 page 114**

Guidelines for Making Responsible Decisions™

You want to eat a snack. You need another serving from the Fruit Group. But you would rather eat some cookies. Answer "yes" or "no" to each of the following questions. Explain each answer

1. Is it healthful to eat cookies instead of fruit?

2. Is it safe to eat cookies instead of fruit?

3. Do you follow rules and laws if you eat cookies instead of fruit?

4. Do you show respect for yourself and others if you eat cookies instead of fruit?

5. Do you follow your family's guidelines if you eat cookies instead of fruit?

6. Do you show good character if you eat cookies instead of fruit?

What is the responsible decision to make?

Vocabulary

Number a sheet of paper from 1–10. Read each definition. Next to each number on your sheet of paper, write the vocabulary word that matches the definition.

nutrient	natural sugar
carbohydrates	food label
table manners	vitamins
Dietary Guidelines	snack
fiber	poultry

1. Meat from chickens, turkeys, or other birds. **Lesson 16**
2. Suggested goals for eating to help you stay healthy and live longer. **Lesson 14**
3. Nutrients that supply the main source of energy for your body. **Lesson 13**
4. Food eaten between meals. **Lesson 15**
5. The part of grains and plant foods that cannot be digested. **Lesson 14**
6. Nutrients that help your body use proteins, carbohydrates, and fats. **Lesson 13**
7. The sugar that is in foods and has not been added. **Lesson 14**
8. A part of a package that lists the ingredients and nutrition information of a food. **Lesson 15**
9. A material in food that is used by the body. **Lesson 13**
10. Polite ways to eat. **Lesson 16**

Health Literacy

Effective Communication

Make a list of ten healthful snacks you enjoy. Trade lists with a friend. Try some of the snacks on your friend's list.

Self-Directed Learning

Find a cookbook that has low-fat recipes. Make a list of five recipes that sound tasty. Make plans with your parents or guardian to make one of the recipes.

Critical Thinking

Answer the following question on a sheet of paper. Why do you need to follow the Dietary Guidelines when you eat at a restaurant?

Responsible Citizenship

Make a poster that shows good table manners. Hang the poster in your school cafeteria.

Multicultural Health

Find a recipe from another country. The recipe should follow the Dietary Guidelines. Ask a parent or guardian to help you make the recipe.

Unit 5

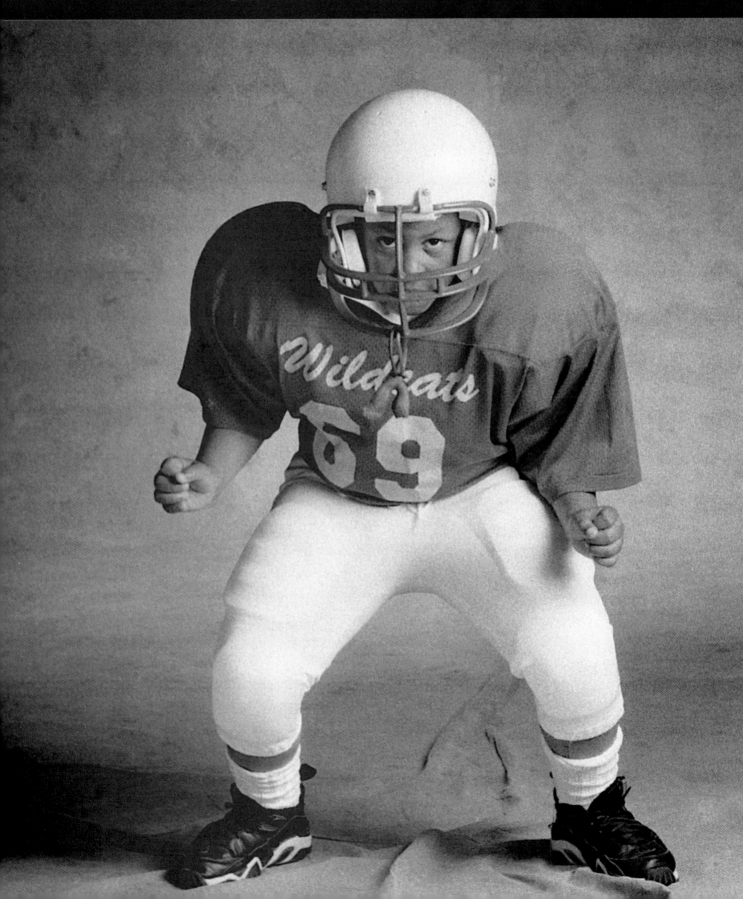

Personal Health
and
Physical Activity

Checkups for Health

Vocabulary

checkup: an examination of your body.

plaque: a sticky material that forms on teeth.

cavity: a hole in the enamel of a tooth.

flossing: a way to remove food and plaque near the gums.

dental floss: a thin thread used to clean teeth.

Life Skills

- I will follow a dental health plan.
- I will have regular checkups.
- I will help my parents or guardian keep my personal health record.

A **checkup** is an examination of your body. Doctors give you checkups to check your health. Dentists give you checkups to look at your teeth. Having regular checkups can help you stay healthy. Your doctor and dentist can help you make a plan for your health.

The Lesson Objectives

- Tell reasons to take care of your teeth.
- Tell ways to remove plaque from your teeth.
- Tell foods and drinks to keep your teeth and gums healthy.
- Make a dental health plan.
- Tell why you need medical checkups.

Why Do I Need to Take Care of My Teeth?

Newborn babies do not have teeth. The first teeth come in after a baby is three months old. A baby goes through a time of teething. Teething means getting teeth. *Primary* (PRY·MEHR·ee) *teeth* are first teeth. Primary teeth are small. They become loose and fall out.

Permanent (PUHR·muh·nuhnt) *teeth* are a second set of teeth. They are also called adult teeth. There are 32 of them. The teeth have different parts.

The *crown* is the part of the tooth that sticks out above the gums. The crown is covered by enamel. *Enamel* is a hard white substance that covers the crown. The *pulp* is the soft inner part of a tooth. The pulp has nerves and blood vessels.

The *root* is the part of the tooth that holds it to the jawbone. The *gums* are the pink tissues around a tooth.

Reasons to Take Care of My Teeth

Your teeth help you look your best. Then you have a nice smile. Clean teeth give you nice breath.

Your teeth help you speak clearly. They work with your tongue to make sounds. Say the word "teeth." Notice how you used your teeth to speak.

Your teeth help you eat. They help you bite and chew. They break up food into smaller pieces.

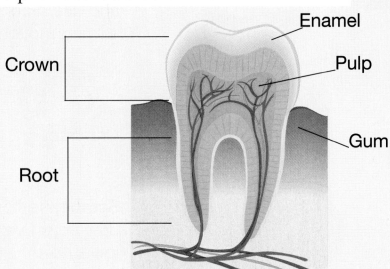

Crown

Enamel

Pulp

Gum

Root

Parts of a Tooth

What Are Ways to Remove Plaque from My Teeth?

Small pieces of food can stick to your teeth. The food mixes with germs in your mouth. This makes plaque. **Plaque** (PLAK) is a sticky material that forms on teeth. Plaque causes tooth decay. Then you can get a cavity. A **cavity** (KA·vuh·tee) is a hole in the enamel of a tooth.

Ways to Remove Plaque from Teeth

• Brush teeth daily.

• Floss your teeth. **Flossing** is a way to remove food and plaque near the gums. **Dental floss** is a thin thread used to floss teeth.

How to Floss Your Teeth

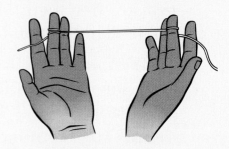

Wind the floss around your middle fingers.

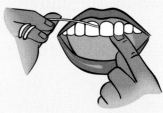

Hold the floss tightly and use a gentle sawing motion.

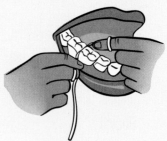

Scrape the floss upward on your lower teeth.

How to Brush Your Teeth

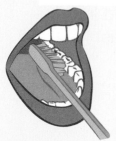

Brush the tops and bottoms of each tooth.

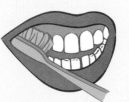

Brush the outside of the teeth gently.

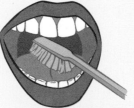

Brush the gums and tongue.

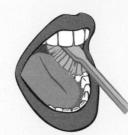

What Foods and Drinks Keep My Teeth and Gums Healthy?

Choose foods and drinks from the Milk, Yogurt, and Cheese Group. They have calcium and vitamin D in them. These foods make the teeth hard. Drink milk. Eat low-fat cheese, cottage cheese, and yogurt.

Choose foods and drinks with vitamin C. Vitamin C helps keep your gums healthy. Eat foods and have drinks that are citrus fruits. Oranges, lemons, and grapefruit are citrus fruits. Eat tomatoes or drink tomato juice. Have tomato soup.

Choose snacks without lots of sugar in them. Eat less sugar to keep from having a cavity. Try vegetables, such as carrot sticks or celery sticks. Try sugar snap peas, or green pepper slices. Eat a piece of fruit. Try an apple or banana. Fruit can satify you when you want something sweet. Have some whole-grain crackers. Put some low-fat dip on them.

Do not eat sticky foods. Cut down on marshmallows and caramels. Give up bubble gum and other gum with sugar in it. Sticky foods and gum with sugar stick to teeth. If you eat them, brush and floss right away.

Dental Health Checklist

1. I brush my teeth at least two times a day.
2. I floss my teeth at least once a day.
3. I limit foods made with sugar.
4. I brush and floss my teeth right after eating foods that have sugar.
5. I eat foods that keep my teeth strong.
6. I eat foods that help keep my gums healthy.
7. I go to the dentist every six months.
8. I wear a mouth-guard when I play sports.
9. I wear a safety belt when I ride in a car.
10. I sit in the back seat when I ride in a car.

Why Do I Need Medical Checkups?

You need a medical checkup to find changes in health. You need to have a medical checkup each year. The doctor checks your body. Some tests might be done. A nurse or doctor will check your height and weight.

Your eyes, ears, nose, and throat are checked. Your heart and lungs are checked. The doctor will check how you are growing. The doctor will ask about your habits.

Your doctor will ask if you have questions. Make a list of questions for your doctor before your checkup. Go over them with your parents or guardian. Your doctor will help you make a health plan.

You need a medical checkup when you have symptoms. The doctor checks you to find out why you are sick. The doctor might do some tests. You might have blood checked. You might have urine checked. You might have your temperature taken. The doctor might give you medicine. You might need to stay home from school.

The doctor will write down facts from your checkup. They are written in a health record. The record is kept by your doctor.

Use Only As Directed

Your doctor might prescribe medicine for you when you are ill. Follow your doctor's directions for taking your medicine. It will not work right if you do not take it the way your doctor says. Finish all your medicine, even if you start to feel better first. Do not give your medicine to anyone else. Do not take medicine a doctor gave to someone else.

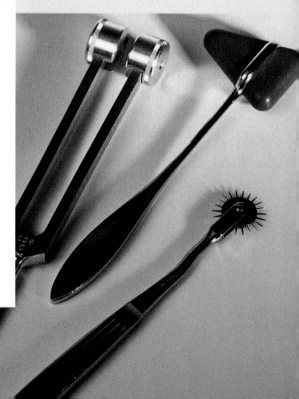

Keep a Health Habits Record

Activity

Life Skill

- I will help my parents or guardian keep my personal health record.

Materials: Spiral notebook, pencil

Directions: Keep notes on your health habits in a small spiral notebook. Take them with you to the doctor.

1. **Write down the physical activities you do.** Tell how often you do them.
2. **Write down the foods and drinks you have for three days.**
3. **Write questions you have for your doctor.** Share your Health Habits Record with your doctor. Make a copy to keep at home.

Lesson 17

Review

Vocabulary

Write a separate sentence using each vocabulary word listed on page 120.

Health Content

1. Why do you need to take care of your teeth? **page 121**
2. What are ways to remove plaque from your teeth? **page 122**
3. What foods and drinks keep your teeth and gums healthy? **page 123**
4. What should be in your dental health plan? **page 123**
5. Why do you need medical checkups? **page 124**

Being Well-Groomed

Vocabulary

grooming: taking care of your body and appearance.

skin: the organ that covers your body.

perspiration: a liquid made in sweat glands.

cuticle: the skin around the nails.

head lice: tiny insects that lay eggs in the hair.

Life Skills

- I will be well-groomed.
- I will get enough rest and sleep.

Grooming is taking care of your body and appearance. You look your best when you are well-groomed. When your body is clean, you keep off germs. You feel good about yourself.

The Lesson Objectives

- Discuss rules for the safe use of grooming products.
- Discuss ways to take care of your clothes.
- Discuss ways to groom your skin and nails.
- Tell grooming products that are used for hair.
- Tell ways to get enough rest and sleep.

What Are Rules for the Safe Use of Grooming Products?

Grooming products are products you use to have a clean body. They are products you use to have a nice appearance. Look in magazines and on TV. You will see ads for grooming products.

Some grooming products are soap, shampoo, toothpaste, and a toothbrush. A hair brush, comb, and hair dryer are grooming products. Perfume and cologne are grooming products.

There are rules for the safe use of grooming products.

- Always ask your parents or guardian before you use a new grooming product.

- Read the label and pay attention to warnings.

- Follow the directions for using a grooming product. Suppose it is for your skin. Try testing the product on a small area first.

- Tell your parents or guardian if you have side effects. A side effect is an unwanted feeling or illness after using a substance. Suppose you get a rash. Suppose your eyes sting. Suppose you itch. These are side effects. Stop using a grooming product if you have side effects.

The Fumes and Mist from Grooming Products

Suppose a person uses nail polish. You can breathe fumes if you are nearby. Suppose someone uses deodorant. You can breathe the mist if you are nearby. Suppose someone uses hairspray. You can breathe the mist if you are nearby. Get near fresh air. Hold your breath until you move away. It can be harmful to breathe in ingredients from them.

Deodorant

Nail Polish

Bath Gel   Lotion

Hairspray

Shampoo   Soap   Bubble Bath

How Can I Take Care of My Clothes?

Read the labels on your clothes. The labels tell directions for caring for the clothes. Some clothes can be washed in cold water only. Some clothes should not go in the dryer. The clothes might be ruined if you do not follow the directions.

Keep your clothes clean. Wash clothes when they become dirty. Tell your parent or guardian if you have a stain on your clothes. The stain might come out if it is cleaned right away.

Keep your clothes in good condition. Hang clothes neatly in a closet. Or fold them neatly in a drawer. Do not toss clothes on the floor. They will wrinkle and be dirty. Fix rips right away. Then they will not get bigger.

Follow family rules for sharing clothes. Ask your parents or guardian the rules for sharing clothes. You might only share clothes with family members. You might have to ask to share clothes with friends. You might have friends clean the clothes before they give them back. You might make a list of clothes you share. Then you will not lose the clothes.

How Can I Groom My Skin?

Skin is the organ that covers your body. Your skin protects your body from harmful rays from the sun. Your skin helps control your body temperature.

Wash your skin each day with soap and water. Washing helps remove dirt, extra oil, and germs. Washing removes perspiration from your skin. **Perspiration** (puhr·spuh·RAY·shuhn) is a liquid made in sweat glands. Perspiration can have an odor. Some people use grooming products for perspiration. An *anti-perspirant* (an·tee·PUHR·spuh·ruhnt) is a product used under the arms to reduce perspiration. A *deodorant* is a product used under the arms to control body odor.

Wash your hands often. Use soap and water. Wash your hands before you eat and after you use the bathroom. Washing hands helps stop the spread of germs.

Use a sunscreen with an SPF of at least 15. The sun can damage your skin. *Sunburn* is a burn on the skin caused by too much sun. SPF is the sun protection factor. A higher SPF number protects your skin longer.

Eat foods with vitamin A. Vitamin A helps keep skin healthy. Green vegetables, orange vegetables, fruits, eggs, and milk contain vitamin A.

Use Skin Products Safely

There are many kinds of skin products for sale. Lotions, bath gels, and perfumes are types of skin products. Ask your parents or guardian before using a new skin product. Check your skin for side effects. Suppose a skin product causes a rash or itching. Stop using the product. Tell your parents or guardian. Some skin products have a very strong scent. Use skin products in small amounts.

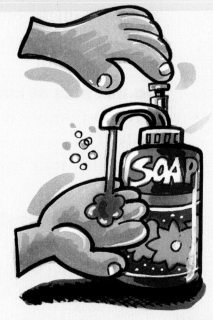

How Can I Groom My Nails?

Your nails protect the ends of your fingers and toes. They are made of hard tissue. The part of the nail you can see is made of dead cells.

You need to groom your nails for good health. Your nails can become dirty and collect germs. They can break. A broken nail can be painful.

Keep your nails clean. Wash your nails with soap and water each day. Scrub your nails with a nail brush. This will clean under the nails.

Trim your nails. There are different ways to trim fingernails. You might clip them. You might file them. Use a nail clipper to trim your toenails. Clip them straight across. You might file the edges.

Do not bite your nails. Germs under the nails might enter your mouth. You might break the nail near the skin. This can be painful.

Do not pick at cuticles. A cuticle (KYOO·ti·kuhl) is the skin around the nails. Germs can enter the skin around the nails. Your fingers can become red and sore.

Keep your nails short when using a computer. Long nails can make it hard to type on a computer keyboard. They can cause you to harm your hands.

Coloring Your Nails

Nail polish is a coating to shine or color nails. Suppose you want to use nail polish. Ask your parent or guardian before you use polish. Do not pick at the nail polish. This can chip your nail. Remove the polish with polish remover. Do not breathe the fumes from nail polish or polish remover.

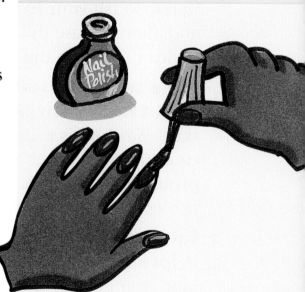

What Are Some Grooming Products for My Hair?

You have about 100,000 hairs on your head. Healthy hair is shiny and clean. Healthy hair helps you have a nice appearance.

Wash your hair often. Use shampoo to wash your hair. Shampoo is a soap that cleans the hair. Choose a shampoo that is right for your hair. Wash your hair correctly. Rub the shampoo into your hair with your fingers. Rinse your hair well. Make sure to rinse all of shampoo out.

You might use a conditioner on your hair. A *conditioner* (kuhn·DI·shuh·nuhr) is a product that helps hair look smooth and shiny. Make sure to rinse all of the conditioner out. Pat your hair dry with a towel. Comb wet hair gently. Your hair might break if you pull it.

You might use a hair dryer. Turn it to the "cool" or "warm" setting. Do not hold it too close to your head. You might burn your skin.

Suppose you want to use other grooming products on your hair. Gel and hair spray are kinds of hair products. Ask your parent or guardian before using a new hair product. Some of these products can harm the eyes. Keep them from your eyes.

Other hair products hold the hair in place. Scrunchies, barrettes, and clips are other hair products. These products should be placed in hair gently. Do not pull or yank them out of hair. Hair might break off.

Hats Off to You!

Some people wear hats to cover their heads. Hats can protect your head from the sun. They can cover a "bad hair day." Do not share hats with other people. This can spread head lice. **Head lice** are tiny insects that lay eggs in the hair. Do not share brushes and combs. This also can spread head lice.

How Can I Get Enough Rest and Sleep?

You need ten to eleven hours of sleep each night. Rest and sleep are important. Your heart beats slower when you rest or sleep. You use less energy. Your body makes new cells. Your body grows.

- Limit foods and drinks that have caffeine. Caffeine is a drug in coffee, chocolate, and tea. Caffeine speeds up what happens in the body. Your heart rate goes up. Your blood pressure goes up. You feel wide awake. It is hard to rest or sleep when you have had caffeine.

- Get plenty of physical activity. This helps you fall asleep at night.

- Plan rest periods during the day. Talk to your teacher if you are tired. You might need to put your head down during recess. Rest after school before you play.

- Have a quiet time before you go to bed. Read or listen to soft music. Take a warm bath. Talk with your parents or guardian. Play with a pet. Unwind and relax.

- Go to sleep at the same time each day. Get up at the same time in the morning.

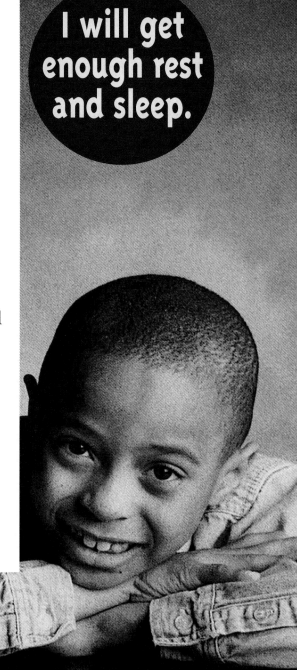

I will get enough rest and sleep.

Use... Guidelines for Making Responsible Decisions™

Situation:

You sleep over at your friend's house. Your hair is a mess when you wake up. Your friend tells you to wear a hat. Your friend gets you a hat from the closet.

Response:

Answer "yes" or "no" to each of the following questions. Explain each answer.

1. Is it healthful to wear your friend's hat?

2. Is it safe to wear your friend's hat?

3. Do you follow rules and laws if you wear your friend's hat?

4. Do you show respect for yourself and others if you wear your friend's hat?

5. Do you follow your family's guidelines if you wear your friend's hat?

6. Do you show good character if you wear your friend's hat?

What is the responsible decision to make?

Lesson 18

Review

Vocabulary

Write a separate sentence using each vocabulary word listed on page 126.

Health Content

1. What are rules for the safe use of grooming products? **page 127**

2. What are ways to take care of your clothes? **page 128**

3. What are ways to groom your skin? Your nails? **pages 129–130**

4. What are some grooming products for your hair? **page 131**

5. What are ways to get enough rest and sleep? **page 132**

Get a Good Workout

Vocabulary

physical fitness: having your body in top condition.

physical fitness plan: a written plan of physical activities you will do.

warm-up: three to five minutes of easy physical activity before a workout.

cool-down: five to ten minutes of easy exercise after a workout.

fitness skills: actions that help you do physical activities.

Life Skill

• **I will get plenty of physical activity.**

Physical activity is moving your muscles. You might enjoy biking or skating. You might enjoy running or swimming. Physical activity helps you have physical fitness. **Physical fitness** is having your body in top condition. Then you are physically fit.

The Lesson Objectives

• Explain why you need to be physically fit.
• List steps to a physical fitness plan.
• Explain how you can work on physical fitness.
• Explain how you can work on fitness skills.

Why Do I Need to Be Physically Fit?

To have good physical health Suppose you are physically fit. Your muscles are firm and strong. You do not tire easily when you play. It is easy for you to carry schoolbooks or groceries. You do not get tired when you climb stairs.

You have energy to play and do things you enjoy. You stay at a healthful weight. Being physically fit helps prevent diseases. Suppose you stay physically fit throughout life. Your heart muscle is strong. Your arteries stay clear of fat. You stay at a healthful weight. This lessens the chance of having heart disease and some cancers.

To get good grades in school Health experts have done research. They learned that regular physical activity helps children do well in school. Your mind is clear. There is good blood flow to your brain.

To get along well with friends Health experts have done other research. They learned that children who are fit are more outgoing. They have more friends with whom they can play. They can enjoy physical activities with other children.

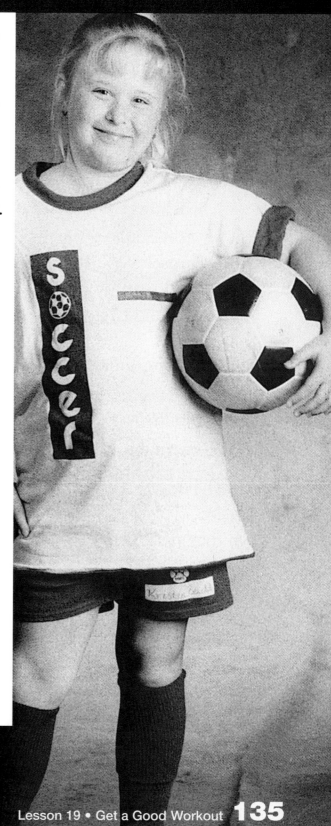

How Do I Make a Physical Fitness Plan?

A **physical fitness plan** is a written plan of physical activities you will do. There are five kinds of physical fitness. Each kind of physical fitness must be in your plan.

- *Heart fitness* is the condition of your heart and blood vessels.

- *Low body fat* is having a lean body without too much fat.

- *Muscle strength* is the ability of your muscles to lift, pull, push, kick, and throw.

- *Muscle endurance* (ihn·DOOR·unts) is the ability to use your muscles for a long time.

- *Flexibility* (flek·suh·BI·luh·tee) is the ability to bend and move easily.

Steps to Make Your Physical Fitness Plan

1. Make a calendar for one week.

2. Make time on three to five days to work on heart fitness and low body fat.

3. Make time on two to four days to work on muscle strength and endurance.

4. Make time on two to three days to work on flexibility.

Plan to Warm Up and Cool Down

A **warm-up** is three to five minutes of easy physical activity before a workout. Walk or jog slowly. This gets your muscles ready for more work. This helps prevent injury to muscles. A **cool-down** is five to ten minutes of easy exercise after a workout.

The rest of this lesson gives physical activities to work on physical fitness.

How Can I Work on Heart Fitness? Low Body Fat?

Heart fitness is the condition of your heart and blood vessels. A strong heart pushes more blood out each time it beats. Between beats, a strong heart has longer to rest.

Aerobic (uhr·OH·bik) exercises are exercises that use a lot of oxygen. They raise your heart beat. You must breathe even when you do them. You must do them for at least twenty minutes. They should be done three to five days a week.

There are many aerobic exercises. Some are swimming, running, and biking. Others are walking, skating, and skiing. These must be done the right way. Suppose you run as fast as you can. You get out of breath and have to stop. This is not aerobic exercise.

You have to get your heart rate up. Then run at a steady pace. You have to keep a steady pace for 20 minutes or more. Slow down if you cannot talk while you run. Slow down if you start to get out of breath.

Aerobic exercises help you have heart fitness. They also help you have low body fat. You keep a neat and trim appearance. You do not get tired easily.

Swim to Work on Heart Fitness

Swim at a steady pace for twenty minutes. You might want to swim laps in a pool. Make sure an adult or lifeguard watches you. Make sure you swim only where it is allowed. Wear goggles to keep chlorine in pool water out of your eyes. Take swimming lessons. The American Red Cross offers them. Learn several strokes. Your arms and legs get a workout. This works on muscle strength. It helps muscle endurance. It helps flexibility, too.

Body Fat Check

Your teacher can help you test your body fat. Your teacher might use skinfold calipers (KA·luh·puhrs). These are used to squeeze the fat on your arm. The thickness tells how much body fat you have.

How Can I Work on Muscle Strength? Muscle Endurance?

Muscle strength is the ability of your muscles to lift, pull, push, kick, and throw. You must use muscles to make them strong. Muscles become weak if you do not use them.

Some exercises make your muscles strong. Climbing a rope makes arm muscles strong. Doing pull-ups makes arm muscles strong. Push-ups make arms strong, too. Riding a bike makes leg muscles strong. Biking makes leg muscles strong.

Sit-ups make the abdomen strong. The abdomen is the part of the body that holds the stomach. Crunches also make the abdomen strong.

Muscle endurance (ihn·DOOR·unts) is the ability to use your muscles for a long time. Suppose you make your bed. You do not use muscles a long time. Suppose you ride your bike a mile to a friend's home. You use your muscles a long time.

Muscle endurance helps you go a distance. Muscle endurance helps you use muscles over and over again. You work on this kind of fitness when you walk or run far. You work on it when you use muscles again and again to ski or skate.

Bike to Work on Muscle Strength and Endurance

Bike for at least 20 minutes without stopping. Ride up and down hills to make leg muscles strong. This builds muscle endurance, too. Biking is best when you can spin your pedals. Talk to your parents or guardian about when and where to ride. Do not ride alone. Learn safety hand signals. Look for bike paths you can use. Wear a helmet and padded gloves. Wear padded shorts, too. Elbow pads and knee pads also can be worn. Keep a water bottle with you.

How Can I Work on Flexibility?

Can you touch your toes? Can you dodge the ball when you play dodge ball? *Flexibility* (flek·suh·BI·luh·tee) is the ability to bend and move easily. This kind of fitness helps you in many ways. You can bend to pick things up. You can move without pulling a muscle.

There are different stretches you can do. Suppose you want to stretch the muscles in your trunk. Stand on your toes. Raise your arms over your head. Stretch your arms as high in the air as you can. When you feel a slight pull, hold the stretch. Count to fifteen.

Plan to stretch different muscle groups. You should work on flexibility two to four days a week. Spend 15 to 30 minutes stretching.

Stretching exercises also can be part of your warm-up. Stretch for a few minutes before aerobic exercises. Stretch before you run or bike. Stretch before you do workouts for muscle endurance. Stretch before you ski or skate.

Dance to Work on Flexibility

Some kinds of dance make flexibility better. Choose ballet or tap dance. Choose modern dance. Try aerobic dance or line dancing. These kinds of dance includes stretches. Make sure to wear the right shoes.

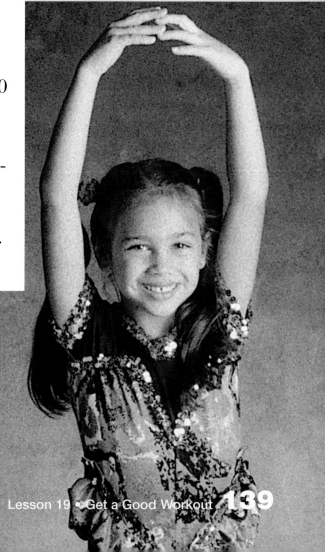

How Can I Work on Fitness Skills?

Fitness skills are skills used to do physical activities.

How to work on agility *Agility* (uh·JI·luh·tee) is the ability to change directions quickly. Play basketball or soccer to work on agility. Play tennis or skip rope.

How to work on balance *Balance* is the ability to keep from falling. Ride your bike to work on balance. Do cartwheels or walk on a balance beam.

How to work on coordination *Coordination* (koh·awr·duh·NAY·shun) is the ability to use more than one body part at a time. One kind is leg to eye coordination. Suppose you want to kick a football. You keep your eye on the football as you let go of it. You move your leg up to kick. Work on coordination. Play soccer or kick ball.

How to work on reaction time *Reaction time* is the time it takes your muscles to respond to a message from your brain. Suppose someone throws a ball for you to catch. It is the time it takes you to get ready to catch the ball.

How to work on speed *Speed* is the ability to move fast. Run fast when you play soccer, football, or baseball.

How to work on power *Power* is the ability to use strong muscles. Kick a ball fast and far. Throw a ball fast and far. Throw a frisbee fast and far.

How Do I Use Fitness Skills?

- To play sports and games
- To perform daily activities
- To move quickly so I will not get hurt

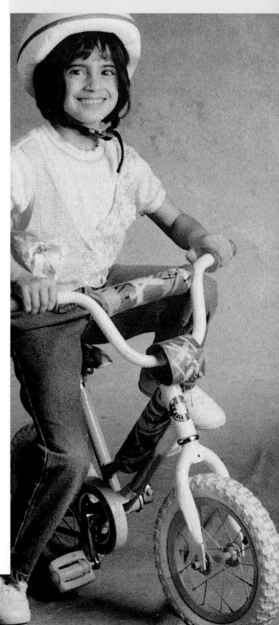

Make a Physical Fitness Plan

Activity

Life Skill

• **I will get plenty of physical activity.**

Materials: Paper, pencil

Directions: Follow the directions below to make a physical fitness plan.

1. **Make a calendar for one week.**
2. **Plan 30 minutes of physical activity on each day of the week.** Write the names of physical activities to work on heart fitness on three to five days. Write the names of physical activities to work on muscle strength and muscle endurance on two to four days. Write the names of physical activities to work on flexibility on two to three days a week.
3. **Plan to do a warm-up and cool-down.**
4. **Follow your physical fitness plan.** Keep track of how much physical activity you get.

Lesson 19

Review

Vocabulary

Write a separate sentence using each vocabulary word listed on page 134.

Health Content

1. Why do you need to be physically fit? **page 135**
2. What are steps to make a physical fitness plan? **page 136**
3. How can you work on heart fitness? Low body fat? **page 137**
4. How can you work on muscle strength? Muscle endurance? Flexibility? **pages 138–139**
5. How can you work on fitness skills? **page 140**

Sporting Safety

Vocabulary

safety equipment: equipment that helps keep you from getting hurt during sports.

mouthguard: an object worn to protect the teeth and gums.

cooperate: to work well with others toward a goal.

Life Skills

- I will follow safety rules for sports and games.
- I will prevent injuries during physical activity.

What sports and games do you enjoy? Do you know the safety rules for them? Always follow safety rules for sports and games. Wear safety equipment. Use good manners. Then you will not get injured. You will keep others safe from injury.

The Lesson Objectives

- Tell ways to keep from getting hurt when you enjoy physical activity.
- Tell how to get ready to take a physical fitness test.
- Tell safety equipment you need for different sports.
- Tell how you can use good manners when you play sports and games.

How Can I Keep from Getting Hurt When I Enjoy Physical Activity?

Physical activity is fun and healthful. But you could be injured if you are not careful.

Follow the rules for the sport or game you are playing. Most sports have rules. These rules are meant to protect you. Do not hit or push other players. Throw balls to other players, not at them. Never aim a ball at another player's head. If you get hurt, do not keep playing. Tell your coach or another responsible adult. They can get you the help you need. You could make an injury worse if you keep playing.

Wear the right clothes, shoes, and equipment for the sport or game you are playing. Many sports have safety equipment. Football, soccer, hockey, baseball, biking, and skating all have special equipment you should wear. This equipment helps keep you from getting hurt. Make sure your equipment is the right size. Your parents or guardian can help you choose the right size. When you buy equipment, the store clerk can help make sure it fits.

Always play in a safe place. Do not play in places where there are harmful objects such as broken glass. Do not play in places where there are people who might harm you. Make sure your parents or guardian know where you will play.

A Watchful Eye

A coach or another responsible adult should watch you play sports. For activities such as biking, make sure there are adults nearby. Do not swim in a place where there are no lifeguards.

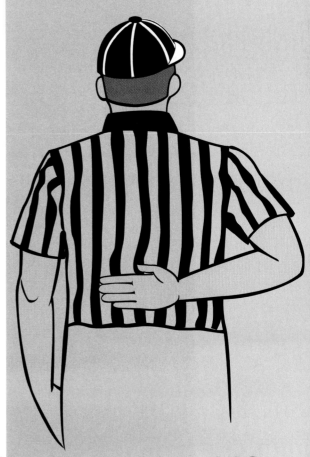

How Can I Get Ready to Take a Physical Fitness Test?

There are two tests to measure physical fitness in boys and girls your age. Practice for the test that will be given at your school.

President's Challenge

- Curl-ups
- Pull-ups
- V-sit and reach
- Shuttle run
- One-mile walk/run

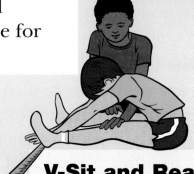

V-Sit and Reach
Measures the flexibility of lower back and calf muscles

Shuttle Run
Measures strength and endurance of leg muscles

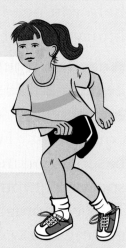

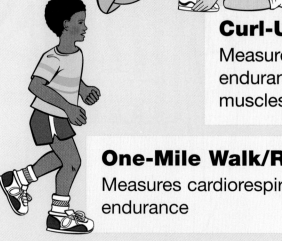

Curl-Ups
Measure strength and endurance of abdominal muscles

One-Mile Walk/Run
Measures cardiorespiratory endurance

Pull-Ups
Measure strength and endurance of upper body muscles

Prudential FITNESSGRAM

- Percent fat
- One-mile walk/run
- Curl-ups
- Push-ups
- Trunk lift
- Sit and reach

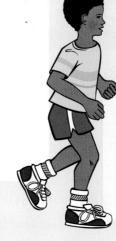

One-Mile Walk/Run
Measures cardio-respiratory endurance

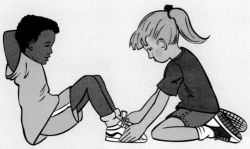

Curl-Ups
Measure strength and endurance of abdominal muscles

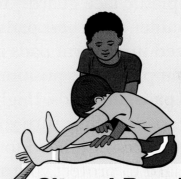

Sit and Reach
Measures the flexibility of lower back and calf muscles

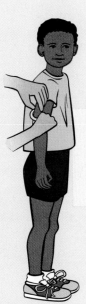

Percent Fat
Measures body composition

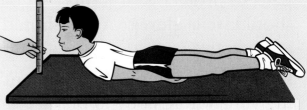

Trunk Lift
Measures strength and flexibility of trunk muscles

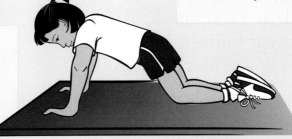
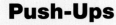

Push-Ups
Measure strength of upper body muscles

What Safety Equipment Do I Need for Sports?

Safety equipment is equipment that helps keep you from getting hurt during sports. You should use safety equipment for any sport or game in which you might get hurt.

Football You should wear a football helmet to play football. This helmet has a strong plastic face guard. You should wear shoulder and chest pads. You might need upper arm pads and elbow pads if you play some positions. You need rib pads, hip pads, thigh pads, and knee pads. Make sure your gear is the right size. You need to wear a mouthguard to protect your teeth. A boy should wear a protective cup.

Soccer You should wear shin guards and a mouthguard when you play soccer. You should wear knee pads and elbow pads to protect your joints. A goalie should wear gloves. A boy should wear a protective cup.

Ice hockey You need equipment covering your whole body to play ice hockey. You must wear a helmet, padded chest and arm guards, shin and knee guards, and gloves. A goalkeeper wears extra equipment such as a face mask. All players should wear mouthguards. A boy should wear a protective cup.

Why You Need a Mouthguard

A **mouthguard** is an object worn to protect the teeth and gums. A mouthguard also can protect your head and jaw. The American Dental Association (ADA) says 13 to 39 percent of tooth injuries happen during sports. Wear a mouthguard during sports where you might fall. Wear a mouthguard during sports where you might be hit in the mouth by a person, ball, or puck.

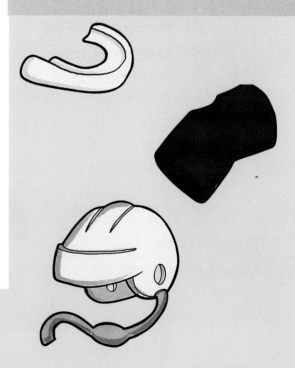

Baseball and softball You should wear a helmet when you bat. The Consumer Product Safety Commission (CPSC) suggests that the helmet have a face guard as well. You might want to wear gloves when you bat. You should wear a leather glove to catch the ball when you play in the infield or outfield. A catcher needs extra gear. This gear includes a face mask, leg guards, and a chest guard. You should wear a mouthguard. A boy should wear a protective cup.

In-line skating Make sure your skates fit well. You need to wear a helmet when you in-line skate. You need wrist guards to protect your wrists when you fall. You need knee pads and elbow pads to protect your joints.

Bicycling Make sure your bike is the right size for you. You need to wear a helmet. Your helmet must fit you well. Wear your helmet down over your forehead. Do not tilt your helmet or wear it on the back of your head. Your bike should have reflectors on the back and front, on the pedals, and on the wheels. You need to keep your pants from catching in your bike wheels. Use a special clip or a rubber band to hold them against your legs. Wear shoes with closed toes when you ride your bike.

Why You Should Wear Safety Glasses

You should think about wearing safety glasses or goggles while playing sports. Many people injure their eyes. For example, many injuries occur when a ball hits the eye. If a ball hits you, it can harm your eye and break the bones around it. Safety glasses or goggles protect the eyes.

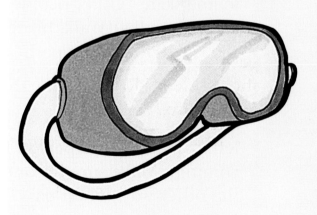

How Can I Use Good Manners When I Play Sports and Games?

To **cooperate** (koh·AH·puh·rayt) is to work well with others toward a goal. Cooperate with others when you enjoy sports and games. Use good manners.

Be a good teammate. You must work as a team for many sports, such as baseball, soccer, and hockey. Team sports help you learn to work well with others. It is good for you to try your best to win. But do not harm others while you play. Be polite to other players on your team and the other team. Do not hit, shove, or kick other players. Follow all the rules.

Use good manners on exercise paths and sidewalks. You might walk, bike, or in-line skate. Other people use the paths and sidewalks. Walk, bike, or skate on the right side of the path. Suppose you are biking or skating on a path. You want to pass someone who is walking ahead of you. Call out, "Passing on your left!" This lets the person know you are coming. Make sure no one is coming the other way. Then pass on the left.

Use good manners at a gym. Let other people exercise in peace. Use only equipment you are allowed to use. Use equipment the way it is meant to be used. Do not make loud noises. Do not block swimming lanes in a pool.

Use Good Manners on the Diving Board

You might enjoy going off the diving board at a pool. Make sure there is no one in the water below you before you jump or dive. Jump or dive straight off the board—not off to the side. Then swim away from the board so other people can use it.

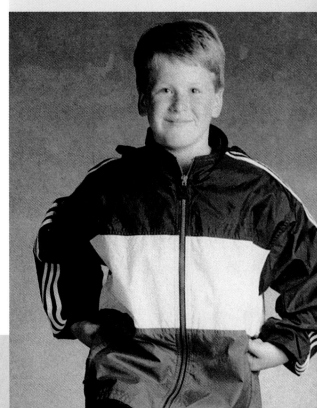

Top Ten List of Ways to Show Respect During Sports and Games

Life Skill

- I will follow safety rules for sports and games.

Materials: Paper, pencil, or markers

Directions: You need to show respect for others during any physical activity.

1. **Write the name of your favorite game or sport at the top of your sheet of paper.**

2. **Write ten ways to show respect for others while playing that game or sport.** Number your list.

3. **Decorate your list using the markers.**

4. **Share your list with your classmates.** If someone else chose the same game or sport, compare lists. Write any new ideas the other person had on the back of your list.

Activity

Lesson 20

Review

Vocabulary

Write a separate sentence using each vocabulary word listed on page 142.

Health Content

1. What are ways you can keep from getting hurt when you enjoy physical activity? **page 143**

2. How can you get ready to take a physical fitness test? **pages 144–145**

3. What exercises are part of each physical fitness test? **pages 144–145**

4. What safety equipment do you need for different sports? **pages 146–147**

5. How can you use good manners when you play sports and games? **page 148**

Unit 5 Review

Health Content

1. Why do you need to take care of your teeth? **Lesson 17 page 121**
2. What health habits should you tell your doctor about? **Lesson 17 page 125**
3. What products can you use for grooming? **Lesson 18 page 127**
4. How much rest and sleep should you get? **Lesson 18 page 132**
5. What are reasons you need to be physically fit? **Lesson 19 page 135**
6. How can you work on muscle endurance? **Lesson 19 page 138**
7. How can you work on flexibility? **Lesson 19 page 139**
8. How can you keep from getting hurt when you enjoy physical activity? **Lesson 20 page 143**
9. What kinds of safety equipment do you need for sports? **Lesson 20 pages 146–147**
10. What are good manners to use when you play sports and games? **Lesson 20 page 148**

Guidelines for Making Responsible Decisions™

Your friend says you do not need to wear a helmet when you ride your bike near your home. Answer "yes" or "no" to each of the following questions. Explain each answer.

1. Is it healthful to wear a bike helmet?
2. Is it safe to wear a bike helmet?
3. Do you follow rules and laws if you wear a bike helmet?
4. Do you show respect for yourself and others if you wear a bike helmet?
5. Do you follow your family's guidelines if you wear a bike helmet?
6. Do you show good character if you wear a bike helmet?

What is the responsible decision to make?

Vocabulary

Number a sheet of paper from 1–10. Read each definition. Next to each number on your sheet of paper, write the vocabulary word that matches the definition.

checkup	cool-down
cavity	grooming
perspiration	cooperate
safety equipment	skin
physical fitness	fitness skills

1. To work well with others toward a goal. **Lesson 20**
2. Equipment that helps keep you from getting hurt during sports. **Lesson 20**
3. The condition of your body. **Lesson 19**
4. A hole in the enamel of a tooth. **Lesson 17**
5. A liquid made in sweat glands. **Lesson 18**
6. Five to ten minutes of easy exercise after a workout. **Lesson 19**
7. Taking care of your body and appearance. **Lesson 18**
8. Actions that help you do physical activities. **Lesson 19**
9. An examination of your body. **Lesson 17**
10. The organ that covers your body. **Lesson 18**

Health Literacy

Effective Communication

Write a poem about ways you can show good manners when you enjoy sports and games. Read your poem for your class.

Self-Directed Learning

Look at the labels of three items of clothing you own. Write down the care instructions on a sheet of paper. Then answer this question. Do you follow the care instructions?

Critical Thinking

Answer the following question on a sheet of paper. Why is it important to wear a mouthguard when you play sports and games?

Responsible Citizenship

Make a poster that shows ways to build each kind of physical fitness. Hang the poster in your school gym.

Family Involvement

Make a physical fitness plan with your family. Include activities your family can enjoy together.

Unit 6

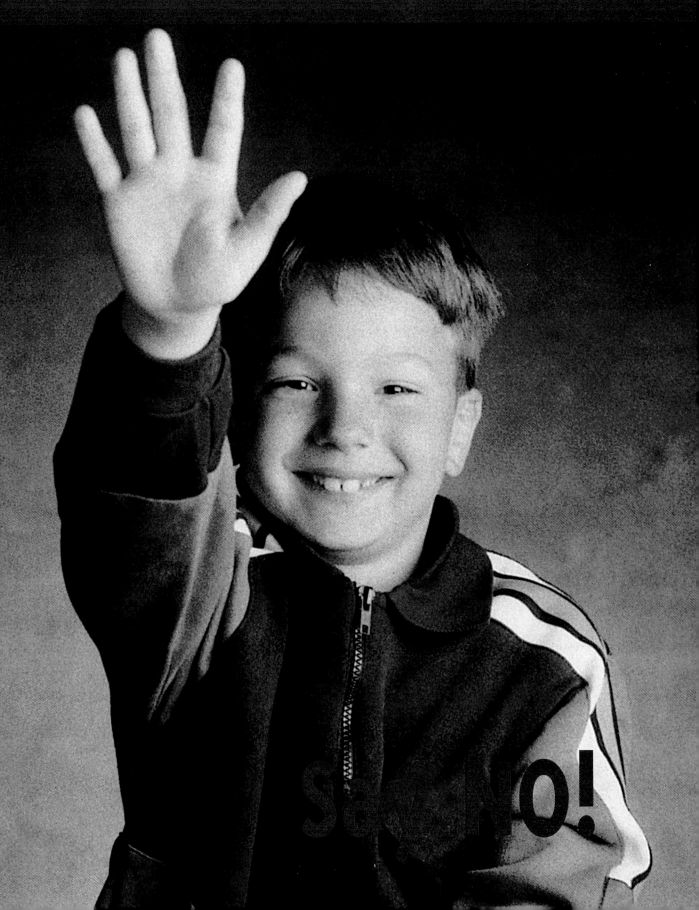

Alcohol, Tobacco, and Other Drugs

Safe Use of Medicines

Vocabulary

drug: a substance that changes how your mind or body works.

medicine: a drug used to treat an illness or injury.

over-the-counter (OTC) medicine: a medicine that you can buy without a doctor's order.

prescription medicine: a medicine that you can buy only if a doctor writes an order.

drug abuse: the unsafe use of a medicine on purpose.

Life Skill

● I will use over-the-counter (OTC) and prescription drugs in safe ways.

Think about the last time you were sick. Your parents or guardian might have given you a medicine. Medicines can be important to your health. But medicines can be harmful if they are not used safely. You need to know how to use medicines safely.

The Lesson Objectives

● Tell how medicines help people.

● Name different kinds of medicines.

● Tell safety rules for using medicines.

● Tell wrong ways to use medicines.

How Do Medicines Help People?

A **drug** is a substance that changes how your mind or body works. There are many kinds of drugs. One kind of drug is a medicine. A **medicine** is a drug used to treat an illness or injury. Medicines can help people in three ways.

A medicine can cure some illnesses. To *cure* is to make well. Suppose you have an earache caused by germs. Your doctor gives you a medicine. The medicine kills the germs. Your earache goes away and you feel better.

A medicine can help the body work the way it should. Suppose a person has diabetes. Diabetes is an illness in which the body cannot use food in normal ways. Medicine helps the body use food in normal ways. But the person is not cured. The person still has diabetes. The person might always have to take medicine.

A medicine can get rid of symptoms. A *symptom* is a change from normal in a person's health. Suppose you have a cold. One of your symptoms is a runny nose. Your parent or guardian might give you a medicine to stop your runny nose. The medicine gets rid of the symptom. But you still have a cold.

How People Take Medicines

- **Swallowing** The medicine might be a tablet, a capsule, or a liquid. An example is cough syrup.

- **Placing on the skin** The medicine might be an ointment, lotion, or shampoo. An example is shampoo for head lice.

- **Breathing** The medicine might be a spray or gas given by a doctor. An example is a gas breathed before surgery to put a patient to sleep.

- **Injecting** Injecting means to use a needle to put medicine through the skin. The medicine might be a vaccine. An example is a tetanus shot.

What Are Kinds of Medicines?

An **over-the-counter (OTC) medicine** is a medicine that you can buy without a doctor's order. You can choose these packages or bottles off the shelf in a store. OTC drugs are sold in drugstores. They also are sold in grocery stores and department stores.

A **prescription** (pri·SKRIP·shuhn) **medicine** is a medicine that you can buy only if a doctor writes an order. It is written for only one person. You cannot choose a prescription medicine off the shelf in a store. You must take the order to a pharmacist. A pharmacist is the person who must prepare the medicine for you. Pharmacists work in drugstores, in hospitals, and in the pharmacies of department stores and grocery stores.

OTC and prescription medicines usually are safe if they are used the right way. They have labels. The label tells how to take the medicine. You also can ask your doctor or pharmacist questions about the medicine. Medicines can be harmful if they are taken the wrong way.

Some Common OTC Drugs

An *analgesic* (a·nuhl·JEE·zik) helps get rid of pain.

An *antacid* helps get rid of stomach upset.

A *decongestant* (DEE·kuhn·JES·tuhnt) helps clear a stuffy nose.

Cough medicine helps stop a cough.

An *antibiotic* (an·ti·by·AH·tik) *ointment* kills germs in cuts and scrapes.

An *allergy* (A·luhr·jee) *medicine* helps itchy eyes and runny noses.

What Are Safety Rules for Taking Medicines?

Follow safety rules for using medicines. The most important rule is:

Take a medicine only from your parents or guardian.

They will tell you if someone else can give you medicine.

There are other safety rules for taking medicines.

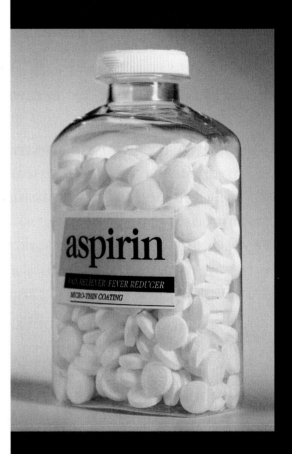

1. Do not take a medicine that is prescribed for someone else.

2. Do not take more medicine than your parent or guardian tells you to take.

3. Do not take medicine more often than your parent or guardian tells you to take it.

4. Do not open a package or bottle of medicine unless it is OK with your parent or guardian. Check for the safety seal. A *safety seal* is an unbroken seal to show a container has not been opened. If the seal is broken, do not use the medicine.

5. Tell your parent or guardian if you have a side effect. A *side effect* is an unwanted feeling or illness after taking a medicine. A side effect might be a rash, an upset stomach, or feeling dizzy. If you have a side effect, your doctor can tell you what to do.

What Are Wrong Ways to Use Medicines?

You should use all medicines the right way. Remember that all medicines are drugs. Drugs change the way your mind or body works. You can be harmed if you do not use a medicine in the right way. There are two wrong ways to use medicines.

One wrong way to use medicine is drug misuse. *Drug misuse* is the unsafe use of a medicine that is not done on purpose. Suppose a person takes the wrong medicine by mistake. This is drug misuse.

Suppose a person does not read a label carefully. The label says to take one tablet every three hours. The person takes three tablets every three hours by mistake. This is drug misuse.

Another wrong way to use medicine is drug abuse. **Drug abuse** is the unsafe use of a medicine on purpose. Suppose a person has a cough. The person should take one teaspoon of a cough medicine. The person takes two teaspoons on purpose. This is drug abuse.

Suppose a person has trouble going to sleep. The person takes a prescription medicine that was prepared for someone else. This is drug abuse.

Drug Addiction

Some medicines can cause drug addiction. *Drug addiction* is being unable to stop using a drug. The person continues to take the drug even if the drug is harmful. The person might get sick in other ways if the drug is stopped. The person might want to stop, but might not know how. Some prescription drugs can cause drug addiction. This is one reason you should not take another person's prescription medicine.

I will use over-the-counter (OTC) and prescription drugs in safe ways.

Use... Guidelines for Making Responsible Decisions™

Situation:

You are at a friend's house. You get a headache. Your friend's older sister says there is medicine in the bathroom cabinet to help your head. She tells you to take two tablets. Your friend says it is OK. He has taken the medicine before.

Response:

Answer "yes" or "no" to each of the following questions. Explain each answer.

1. Is it healthful to take the medicine?
2. Is it safe to take the medicine?
3. Do you follow rules and laws if you take the medicine?
4. Do you show respect for yourself and others if you take the medicine?
5. Do you follow your family's guidelines if you take the medicine?
6. Do you show good character if you take the medicine?

What is the responsible decision to make?

Lesson 21

Review

Vocabulary

Write a separate sentence using each vocabulary word listed on page 154.

Health Content

1. What are ways medicines help people? **page 155**
2. What are different kinds of medicines? **page 156**
3. Who should give you medicines? **page 157**
4. What are safety rules for taking medicines? **page 157**
5. What are wrong ways to use medicines? **page 158**

Say NO to Alcohol

Vocabulary

alcohol: a drug found in some beverages that slows down the body.

cancer: a disease in which harmful cells grow.

heart disease: a disease of the heart and blood vessels.

Life Skill

● I will not drink alcohol.

Alcohol is a drug found in some beverages that slows down the body. It is against the law for someone your age to drink alcohol. Alcohol harms the mind and body. You will learn ways alcohol is harmful. You will learn why you should choose not to drink alcohol.

The Lesson Objectives

● Explain how drinking alcohol harms the mind.

● Describe how drinking alcohol harms the body.

● Explain how drinking alcohol harms the community.

● Tell ways to say NO to drinking alcohol.

How Does Alcohol Harm the Mind?

Alcohol changes the way the brain works. It slows down the brain. The mind does not work as well if a person drinks alcohol. A person might not be in control of what he or she does.

Alcohol can cause people to make wrong decisions. People who drink alcohol might make decisions that are not responsible. They might make decisions that are unsafe. Their decisions might lead to accidents.

Alcohol can cause people to let out feelings in harmful ways. People who have been drinking alcohol might say things they would not normally say. They might hit someone if they are angry. They might say something mean. They might not think about what could happen if they do or say mean things.

Alcohol can cause people to forget things. People who have been drinking alcohol might not remember things they have learned. They might have a hard time learning new things.

Alcohol can cause people to feel sad. People who have been drinking alcohol might think their problems are worse than they are. They might feel bad about themselves.

Drinking Alcohol Harms the Whole Body

When someone drinks alcohol, the alcohol goes to the stomach. But it is not digested like food. Alcohol passes quickly out of the stomach and small intestine and into the bloodstream. It moves through the bloodstream to all body cells. It goes through the blood to the brain.

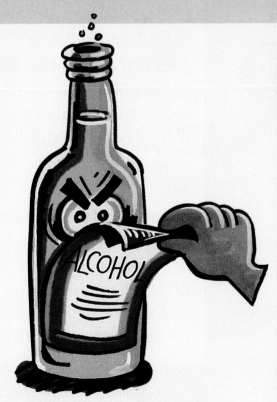

How Does Alcohol Harm the Body?

Alcohol causes the brain to slow down. The brain controls every organ in the body. The brain controls all the body systems. The body does not work right if a person drinks alcohol. The person cannot control his or her body.

Alcohol can cause people to lose control of their muscles. The brain controls the muscles. Alcohol slows down the brain. Muscles do not work together the way they should. People slow down. They cannot move quickly.

When this happens, people cannot walk straight. They cannot speak clearly because the tongue is a muscle. Things look blurry because eye muscles do not work together.

Alcohol can cause people to have accidents. People trip and fall because they cannot walk straight. They run into things because they cannot see well. They might not see traffic coming when they cross a street.

Alcohol can cause people to feel less pain. When people who have been drinking alcohol are injured, they do not feel as much pain. They do not know they have been injured. They might not know if they need help.

Alcohol Causes Diseases

A person who drinks alcohol for a long time can get diseases. Alcohol can cause cancers of the liver, mouth, voice box, and stomach. **Cancer** is a disease in which harmful cells grow. Alcohol can cause heart disease. **Heart disease** is a disease of the heart and blood vessels.

I will not drink alcohol.

How Can Drinking Alcohol Harm the Community?

A person who drinks alcohol is not the only person who is harmed. Other people who do not drink alcohol can be harmed. The people in your town can be harmed by alcohol. They can be harmed even if they do not drink alcohol. There are three ways alcohol can harm the community.

Alcohol can cause accidents. Many car crashes are caused by drivers who have been drinking alcohol. Many fires are started by people who have been drinking alcohol. They do not know what they are doing when they have been drinking.

Alcohol can cause crime and violence. Many crimes are committed by people who are drinking alcohol. Many people who are in prison were drinking alcohol at the time they committed a crime. They were not in control of their behavior. They let out their feelings in harmful ways.

Alcohol can cause problems between family members. A family member who drinks alcohol can harm other family members. The person who drinks alcohol might argue with other family members. The person might break promises to family members.

If Someone Close to You Has a Drinking Problem

Suppose someone close to you has a drinking problem. This person drinks alcohol often or drinks a lot at one time. You might feel guilty. You might think the person drinks alcohol because you have done something wrong. You might feel upset. You might not know how this person will act. You might feel shame. You might try to hide your feelings.

You can talk to someone if this is happening to you. Talk to a parent, a guardian, or another trusted adult. Talk to your school counselor.

What Do I Choose When I Do Not Drink Alcohol?

When you choose not to drink alcohol, you choose these things instead.

I choose to keep my mind clear. I want to remember things. I want to make responsible decisions.

I choose to keep my body working right. I want to walk and talk normally. I want to move quickly. I want to keep from having accidents.

I choose good character. I want to be honest with my family. I want to follow my family's guidelines.

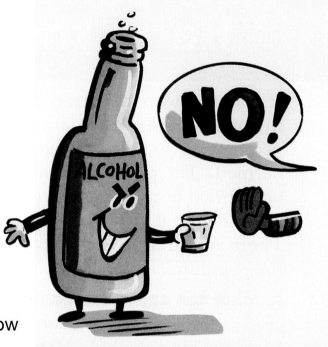

I'm Choosy!

Activity

Life Skill

• **I will not drink alcohol.**

Materials: Paper and pencil

Directions: Complete this activity to think of reasons not to drink alcohol.

1. **Think of something you like to do.** Write it down. You might write, "I like to play board games."

2. **Write down what would happen if you drank alcohol before the activity.** You might write, "I could not play well because alcohol slows down the brain."

3. **Read what you like to do out loud.** Then read what would happen if you drank alcohol. Then say, "I'm choosy! I choose not to drink alcohol."

Resistance Skills

1. Say NO in a firm voice.

2. Give reasons for saying NO.

3. Match your actions with your words.

4. Keep away from situations in which peers might try to talk you into wrong decisions.

5. Keep away from peers who make wrong decisions.

6. Tell an adult if someone tries to talk you into a wrong decision.

7. Help your friends to make responsible decisions.

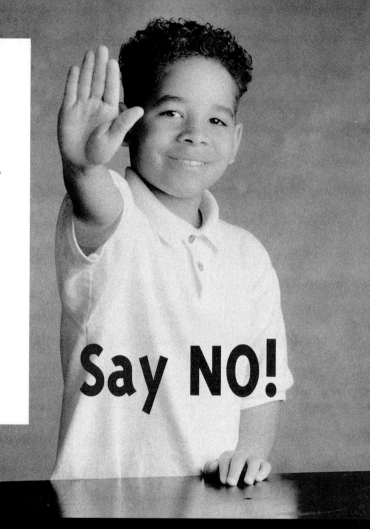

Say NO!

Lesson 22

Review

Vocabulary

Write a separate sentence using each vocabulary word listed on page 160.

Health Content

1. What are ways alcohol harms the mind? **page 161**

2. What are ways alcohol harms the body? **page 162**

3. What are ways drinking alcohol harms the community? **page 163**

4. What do you choose when you do not drink alcohol? **page 164**

5. What are ways you can say NO to drinking alcohol? **page 165**

Say NO to Tobacco

Vocabulary

tobacco: a plant that contains chemicals that are harmful to health.

nicotine: a drug in tobacco that speeds up the body.

tar: a brown, sticky substance in tobacco that is harmful.

smokeless tobacco: tobacco that is not burned.

secondhand smoke: the smoke from other people's cigarettes and cigars.

Life Skills

● **I will not use tobacco.**

● **I will protect myself from secondhand smoke.**

Tobacco (tuh·BA·koh) is a plant that contains chemicals that are harmful to health. When a person smokes or chews tobacco, the chemicals get into the body. Some of these chemicals are drugs. You will learn how tobacco harms the body. You will learn why you should not use tobacco.

The Lesson Objectives

● Tell how smoking harms health.

● Tell how smokeless tobacco harms health.

● Tell how secondhand smoke harms health.

● Tell how tobacco use can change the way a person looks.

● Tell ways to say NO to using tobacco.

How Does Smoking Harm Health?

Some people smoke tobacco in cigarettes, cigars, and pipes. Smoking harms health in three ways.

Smoking causes heart disease.
Tobacco contains the harmful drug nicotine. **Nicotine** (NI·kuh·teen) is a drug in tobacco that speeds up the body. Nicotine in smoke enters the lungs. It passes into the blood and then to other parts of the body.

Nicotine makes the heart beat faster than it should. Then the heart is working harder than it should. Nicotine causes the blood vessels to become narrow. Blood does not flow as easily to the heart. A person who smokes can have a heart attack.

Smoking causes cancer. Tobacco contains chemicals that can cause cancer. One of these chemicals is tar. **Tar** is a brown, sticky substance in tobacco that is harmful. Tar coats the air passages in the lungs. It damages the lungs. A person who smokes can get lung cancer.

Smoking causes breathing problems.
Some chemicals in tobacco can cause a person to get out of breath. The person cannot do everyday activities without getting tired.

Addiction to Nicotine

Nicotine is very addictive (A·DIK·tiv). This means that a person who uses tobacco gets used to having nicotine in the body. The person cannot get along without it. It is very hard to quit. Many people who try to quit using tobacco go back to using it. Do not start using tobacco. You can get addicted to nicotine right away. This means you can get addicted if you try just one cigarette, one cigar, or one chew.

I will not use tobacco.

I will not use tobacco.

How Does Smokeless Tobacco Harm Health?

Smokeless tobacco is tobacco that is not burned. It is chewed or placed between the cheek and the gums. Smokeless tobacco harms health in four ways.

Smokeless tobacco causes heart disease. The nicotine from smokeless tobacco gets into the bloodstream. It causes blood vessels to narrow. A person who uses smokeless tobacco can have a heart attack.

Smokeless tobacco causes cancer. The chemicals in smokeless tobacco cause cancer of the cheeks, gums, tongue, and throat. Chemicals get into saliva. The saliva is swallowed. The chemicals go to the digestive system. The chemicals cause cancer.

Smokeless tobacco causes gum disease. The gums turn red. They swell and bleed. Teeth get loose and fall out.

Smokeless tobacco can cause ulcers. An ulcer is an open sore. A person who uses smokeless tobacco gets ulcers in the mouth. The person's saliva contains chemicals. The saliva is swallowed and goes to the stomach. The person gets ulcers in the stomach.

Not Sugar Free

Tobacco tastes bad. So the people who sell smokeless tobacco add sugar and flavoring. The sugar can cause tooth decay. A person who uses smokeless tobacco can get cavities. Smokeless tobacco also contains gritty or sandy materials. These materials wear down the teeth. Cavities and wearing down of teeth do not take years to happen. They happen to children and teens.

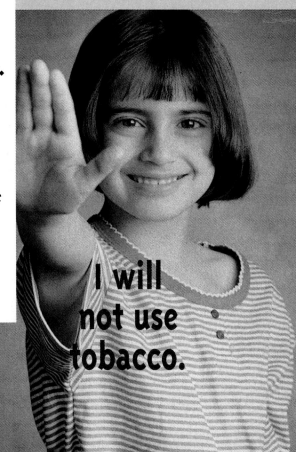

I will not use tobacco.

How Does Secondhand Smoke Harm Health?

Secondhand smoke is the smoke from other people's cigarettes and cigars. This smoke is harmful to people who do not smoke. The people who do not smoke still breathe the smoke. Secondhand smoke harms health in three ways.

Secondhand smoke causes cancer. A person who breathes secondhand smoke gets harmful chemicals in his or her body. These chemicals cause lung cancer.

Secondhand smoke causes more respiratory illnesses. A person who breathes secondhand smoke might get more colds and flu. A person might get asthma. *Asthma* (AZ·muh) is a condition in which the air passages become narrow. People who have asthma can have a hard time breathing.

Secondhand smoke affects the eyes. Smoke makes a person's eyes itch and sting. The eyes might water and get red.

Many public places have banned smoking because of secondhand smoke. Tell your parents or guardian if you see someone smoking in a no-smoking business or area.

Healthful Friends Don't Smoke or Chew

Using tobacco can harm friendships. Healthful friendships are important for good health. Most children, teens, and adults do not use tobacco. They want friends who do not use tobacco. They want friends who take care of their health. They want friends who follow family guidelines.

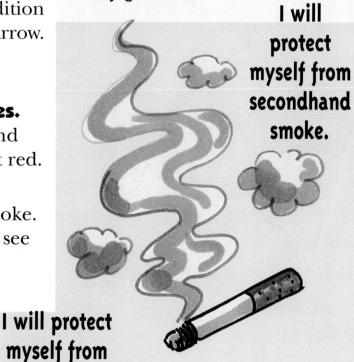

I will protect myself from secondhand smoke.

I will protect myself from secondhand smoke.

No-Tobacco Ad

Activity

Life Skill

- **I will not use tobacco.**

Materials: Magazines, scissors, poster paper, glue or tape

Directions: Read what is inside the box. Follow the steps to make your own ad.

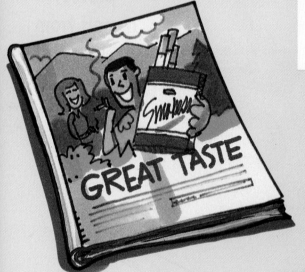

Tobacco Ads

Some ads try to sell tobacco. An ad is a way of selling something. You see ads that sell tobacco in magazines and on billboards along the highway.

There is a tiny box in the corner of each ad. The box has a message. The message gives one way tobacco harms health. The message is very small. It does not give all the ways tobacco harms health.

1. **Look through magazines.** Think about how you can use pictures to make your own ad. Your ad should try to get people NOT to use tobacco.

2. **Cut out pictures to use in your ad.** Glue the pictures on a piece of poster paper.

3. **Write three ways using tobacco is harmful.** Make the letters big.

4. **Display your ad in your classroom.**

How Can Tobacco Use Change the Way a Person Looks?

Using tobacco turns teeth yellow. It turns fingernails yellow. Tobacco causes a person's face to wrinkle at a young age. Even teens who smoke start to get wrinkles.

Smokeless tobacco causes teeth to get stained yellow and brown. Teeth begin to fall out. It does not take long for this to happen. This happens to young people.

Smokeless tobacco causes people to spit. Spitting out tobacco disgusts other people.

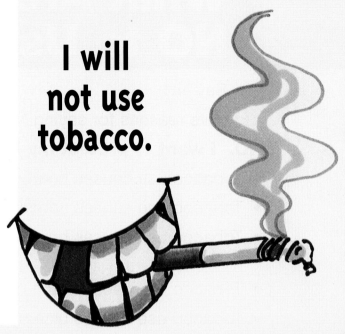

I will not use tobacco.

Tobacco Is Out of Fashion

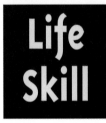

Life Skill

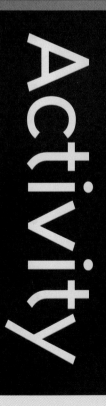

Activity

● **I will not use tobacco.**

Materials: Magazines, scissors, black markers, brown markers, yellow markers

Directions: Show how tobacco use can change the way a person looks.

1. **Find magazine pictures of people who look healthy.** Pretend the people use tobacco.

2. **Use the markers to color the teeth and fingernails of the people in the magazine pictures.** For example, you might color a tooth black to show it is missing. You might use the yellow and brown markers to put stains on the teeth. You might put wrinkles on the skin.

3. **Write on the pictures, "How People Who Use Tobacco REALLY Look."**

What Are Ways to Say NO to Using Tobacco?

1. Say NO.

2. Give reasons for saying NO.

NO. I want to protect my health.

- Tobacco use causes heart disease.
- Tobacco use causes cancer.
- Tobacco use causes breathing problems.
- Tobacco use causes gum disease.
- Tobacco use causes ulcers.

NO. I want to stay safe.

- Lighted tobacco products can start fires.
- Using tobacco while doing something else can cause accidents.

NO. I want to follow rules and laws.

- The sports team I am on has rules against tobacco.
- My school has a no-smoking rule.

NO. I want to show respect for myself and others.

- I do not want others to breathe secondhand smoke.
- I do not want others to see me spit out tobacco

NO. I want to follow my family's guidelines.

NO. I want to show good character.

3. Match your actions with your words.

4. Keep away from situations in which peers might try to get you to use tobacco.

5. Keep away from peers who smoke.

6. Tell an adult if someone tries to get you to smoke or buy tobacco.

7. Help your friends decide not to use tobacco.

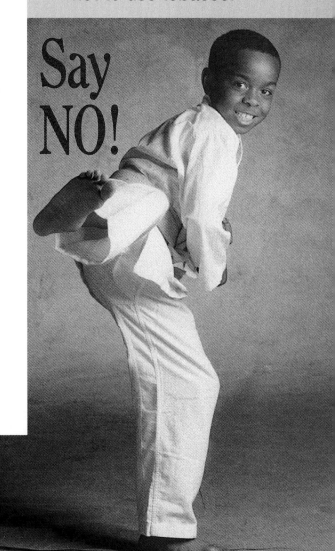

Say NO!

Use... Guidelines for Making Responsible Decisions™

Situation:

You are at your uncle's house. Your uncle smokes cigars. Your cousin sneaks a cigar. Your cousin tries to talk you into putting it in your mouth. She says, "We won't light it. We'll just pretend to smoke it. It won't hurt us."

Response:

Answer "yes" or "no" to each of the following questions. Explain each answer.

1. Is it healthful to put a cigar in your mouth?
2. Is it safe to put a cigar in your mouth?
3. Do you follow rules and laws if you put a cigar in your mouth?
4. Do you show respect for yourself and others if you put a cigar in your mouth?
5. Do you follow your family's guidelines if you put a cigar in your mouth?
6. Do you show good character if you put a cigar in your mouth?

What is the responsible decision to make?

Lesson 23

Review

Vocabulary

Write a separate sentence using each vocabulary word listed on page 166.

Health Content

1. What are ways smoking harms health? **page 167**
2. What are ways smokeless tobacco harms health? **page 168**
3. What are ways secondhand smoke harms health? **page 169**
4. What does using tobacco do to a person's looks? **page 171**
5. What are ways to say NO to using tobacco? **page 172**

Unit 6

Lesson 24

Say NO to Illegal Drugs

Vocabulary

illegal drugs: drugs that are against the law.

inhalant: a chemical that is breathed.

marijuana: a drug that harms memory and concentration.

stimulant: a drug that speeds up body functions.

depressant: a drug that slows down body functions.

Life Skills

- I will not be involved in illegal drug use.
- I will say NO if someone offers me a harmful drug.
- I will tell ways to get help for someone who uses drugs in harmful ways.

Illegal drugs are drugs that are against the law. These drugs harm health. People can be harmed soon after they take the drug. People can be harmed if they take the drug for a long time.

The Lesson Objectives

- Tell ways inhalants harm health.
- Tell ways marijuana harms health.
- Tell ways stimulants and depressants harm health.
- Tell ways to say NO to abusing drugs.
- Tell ways you can stop drug abuse.

How Can Inhalants Harm Health?

An **inhalant** (in·HAY·luhnt) is a chemical that is breathed. Some inhalants are everyday products.

Household cleaners and paint thinners are inhalants. These products give off fumes or gases. The fumes can be harmful if a person breathes too much of them at one time. The fumes can be harmful if a person breathes a little of them for a long time.

Inhalants can harm health right now. People who breathe harmful fumes can get sick right away. They might get dizzy. They might get headaches. Their heart might beat faster. They might have trouble breathing. They might vomit.

Inhalants can harm health later. Suppose a person uses products that give off harmful fumes for weeks or months. The person does not get fresh air when using the products.

Body organs can be damaged. The brain, liver, kidneys, and heart can be harmed. Brain cells can die. The person might have trouble learning. Muscles can be affected. The person might have trouble coordinating muscles. Cells can be changed. The person might get cancer.

Use Care! Get Air!

Always get fresh air when you use a product that gives off fumes. Use these products only when an adult is there.

Inhalants That Are Medicines

Some medicines are sold as inhalants. A doctor prescribes the medicine. The person breathes the medicine into the body. A person who has asthma might use an inhalant. This person might use an inhaler to take it. An *inhaler* (in·HAY·luhr) is a device that sprays medicine into a person's air passages.

How Can Marijuana Harm Health?

Marijuana (mer·uh·WAH·nuh) is a drug that harms memory and concentration. Concentration is how long a person is able to pay attention to something. It is against the law in most places to use marijuana. Marijuana usually is smoked. The chemicals in marijuana go to the lungs and then to the bloodstream. The chemicals go to all parts of the body. Marijuana can harm health in these ways.

Marijuana can harm health right now.

People who use marijuana cannot remember things. They cannot learn new things. They cannot see things well. They cannot coordinate their muscles. They are clumsy and have accidents.

Marijuana can cause people to see things that are not real. People feel sad for no reason. They feel mixed up. They cannot think clearly. They make poor decisions. They say and do things they would not do normally.

Marijuana can harm health later.

People who use marijuana for a long time stop caring about anything. They lose interest in family and friends. They do not want to play sports or do other things. Marijuana can cause cancer and heart disease.

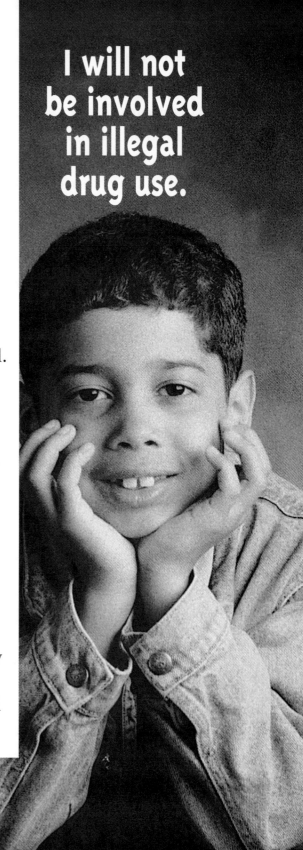

I will not be involved in illegal drug use.

How Can Stimulants Harm Health?

A **stimulant** (STIM·yuh·luhnt) is a drug that speeds up body functions. Some stimulants are medicines. They are okay to use if a doctor prescribes them.

Stimulants can be harmful if they are used in wrong ways on purpose. This is called drug abuse. A wrong way to use stimulants is to take stimulants prescribed for someone else. Abuse of stimulants can harm health in these ways.

Stimulants can harm health right now.

People who abuse stimulants get cranky and jumpy. They get dizzy. They lose their appetite. They cannot sleep.

Stimulants can harm health later.

People who abuse stimulants for a long time might feel upset all the time. They feel very sad for no reason. They might see things that are not real.

Cocaine (koh·KAYN) is a stimulant made from the leaves of the coca bush. It is against the law to use cocaine. Cocaine is very dangerous. Cocaine can cause the heart to stop working. A person who uses cocaine can die right away. Crack is a stimulant that is stronger than cocaine. It is illegal and very dangerous.

Stay Away from Drug Abusers

People who use cocaine and crack are drug abusers. They become addicted. They have to have these drugs. They might commit crimes to get money to buy drugs. They might rob and hurt people to get money. Stay away from people who sell or use cocaine or crack. They might be dangerous.

I will say NO if someone offers me a harmful drug.

How Can Depressants Harm Health?

A **depressant** (di·PRE·suhnt) is a drug that slows down body functions. Some depressants are medicines. They are okay to use if a doctor prescribes them. Depressants can be harmful if they are used the wrong way. This is drug abuse. Abusing depressants can harm health.

Ways depressants can harm health right now. People who abuse depressants can have trouble breathing. They have trouble speaking. They get very sleepy and might not be able to wake up.

Ways depressants can harm health later. People who abuse depressants can get addicted. They cannot stop using the drugs.

Use... Guidelines for Making Responsible Decisions™

Situation:

You are at a friend's house. The friend wants to paint a stool for her mother's birthday. She paints the stool in her bedroom closet with the door closed.

Response:

Answer "yes" or "no" to each of the following questions. Explain each answer.

1. Is it healthful to paint inside a closet?
2. Is it safe to paint inside a closet?
3. Do you follow rules and laws if you paint inside a closet?
4. Do you show respect for yourself and others if you paint inside a closet?
5. Do you follow your family's guidelines if you paint inside a closet?
6. Do you show good character if you paint inside a closet?

What is the responsible decision to make?

My Drug-Free Pledge

If someone offers a pill or drink,
I never have to stop and think.
I can resist—the way I know
Is use a firm voice for saying NO!

When I say NO! to harmful drugs,
I make my voice be heard.
I let them know I won't. I match
My actions with my words.

If someone tells me I'll be hip
If I take a puff or take a sip,
I can resist—the way I know
Is give good reasons for saying NO!

To keep myself from being hurt,
And stay healthy every day,
I always keep myself alert
And from drugs just stay away!

If someone tells my friend to try
Illegal drugs, I'll tell her why
She can resist—the way I know
Is help my family and friends say NO!

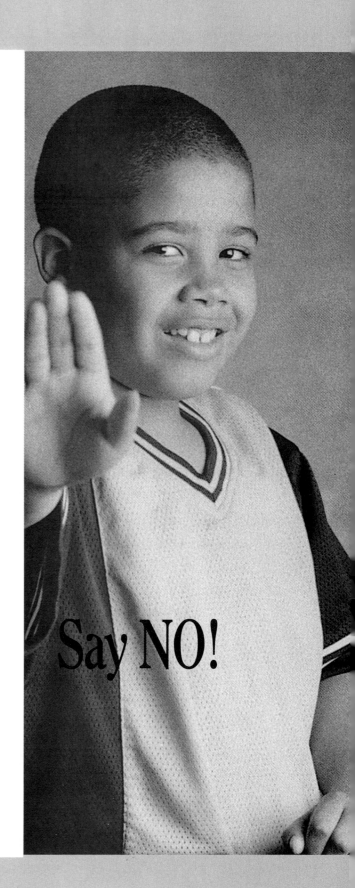

Say NO!

How Can I Help Stop Drug Abuse?

You can help stop drug abuse in two ways.

You can tell your parents, guardian, or another trusted adult if a friend tries drugs. Adults can get help for your friend. There are many people who can help people who abuse drugs. The school counselor can help. Doctors and nurses can help. Sometimes people who abuse drugs go to special hospitals or clinics. The people who work there know how to treat people who are addicted to drugs.

You can help keep your friends from trying drugs. Help your friends make responsible decisions. Make a promise to your friends that you will not abuse drugs. Have your friends promise you and each other that they will not abuse drugs. Promise you will care about one another.

Many times friends do things because other friends do them. You can stick together and choose not to abuse drugs. You can stay away from illegal drug use.

Be a True Friend

Suppose a friend starts to talk about using drugs. Be a true friend. Tell that person you care about him or her. Tell that person you want him or her to be healthy. Tell a trusted adult if you think a friend is using drugs. Your friend might get angry at you. But you are doing the right thing. You are showing you care about your friend. Your friend will thank you later.

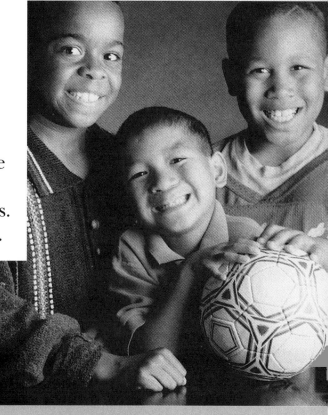

Did You Know...?
Caffeine Is a Drug

Caffeine is a stimulant found in chocolate and some beverages. Too much caffeine can keep a person awake at night. It can make a person cranky and jumpy. It can cause headaches and stomachaches. Limit the amount of chocolate you eat. Limit beverages that have caffeine. Look for labels on soda pops that say "Decaffeinated" or "No caffeine."

Caffeine Surprise!

You might think it is okay to drink bottled water. But some bottled water has caffeine added. Read the labels on bottled water. If a bottle of water has caffeine, the label will tell you.

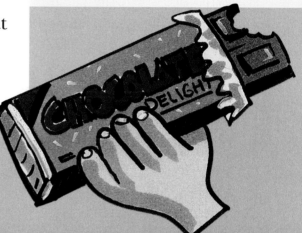

Lesson 24

Review

Vocabulary

Write a separate sentence using each vocabulary word listed on page 174.

Health Content

1. What are two ways inhalants can harm health? **page 175**
2. What are two ways marijuana can harm health? **page 176**
3. What are two ways stimulants can harm health? Two ways depressants can harm health? **pages 177–178**
4. What are ways to say NO to drugs? **page 179**
5. What are ways you can help stop drug abuse? **page 180**

Unit 6 Review

Health Content

1. How do medicines help people?
   Lesson 21 page 155

2. Who are the only people who should give you medicine?
   Lesson 21 page 157

3. What is an example of drug misuse? **Lesson 21 page 158**

4. How does alcohol harm the body? **Lesson 22 page 162**

5. What are ways to say NO to drinking alcohol? **Lesson 22 page 165**

6. How does smokeless tobacco harm health? **Lesson 23 page 168**

7. How might using tobacco change a person's looks?
   Lesson 23 page 171

8. How can abusing inhalants harm health? **Lesson 24 page 175**

9. How can marijuana harm health?
   Lesson 24 page 176

10. What should you tell a person who tries to get you to use drugs? **Lesson 24 page 179**

Guidelines for Making Responsible Decisions™

An older student lives next to you. He says he knows a shortcut home from school. He takes you down an alley. He says teens are using crack there. He says they will not bother you. Answer "yes" or "no" to each of the following questions. Explain each answer.

1. Is it healthful to go near people who are using drugs?

2. Is it safe to go near people who are using drugs?

3. Do you follow rules and laws if you go near people who are using drugs?

4. Do you show respect for yourself and others if you go near people who are using drugs?

5. Do you follow your family's guidelines if you go near people who are using drugs?

6. Do you show good character if you go near people who are using drugs?

What is the responsible decision to make?

Vocabulary

Number a sheet of paper from 1–10. Read each definition. Next to each number on your sheet of paper, write the vocabulary word that matches the definition.

stimulant	nicotine
prescription medicine	cancer
smokeless tobacco	inhalant
drug	alcohol
depressant	tar

1. A drug in tobacco that speeds up the body. **Lesson 23**
2. A disease in which harmful cells grow. **Lesson 22**
3. A chemical that is breathed. **Lesson 24**
4. A drug found in some beverages that slows down the body. **Lesson 22**
5. A substance that changes how your mind or body works. **Lesson 21**
6. Tobacco that is chewed or placed between the cheek and the gums. **Lesson 23**
7. A drug that speeds up body functions. **Lesson 24**
8. A medicine that you can buy only if a doctor writes an order. **Lesson 21**
9. A brown, sticky substance in tobacco that is harmful. **Lesson 23**
10. A drug that slows down body functions. **Lesson 24**

Health Literacy

Effective Communication

Suppose a classmate dares you to smoke a cigarette. What would you say to your classmate?

Self-Directed Learning

Go to a grocery store. Look at the labels on soda pop. List five soda pops that have caffeine. List five soda pops that do not have caffeine.

Critical Thinking

Draw a picture of a person. Show how the person's body might be harmed by drinking alcohol.

Responsible Citizenship

Write a safety rule for taking medicines on an index card. Tape the card to the cabinet where your family keeps medicines.

Family Involvement

Practice with your parents or guardian how to say NO to drugs.

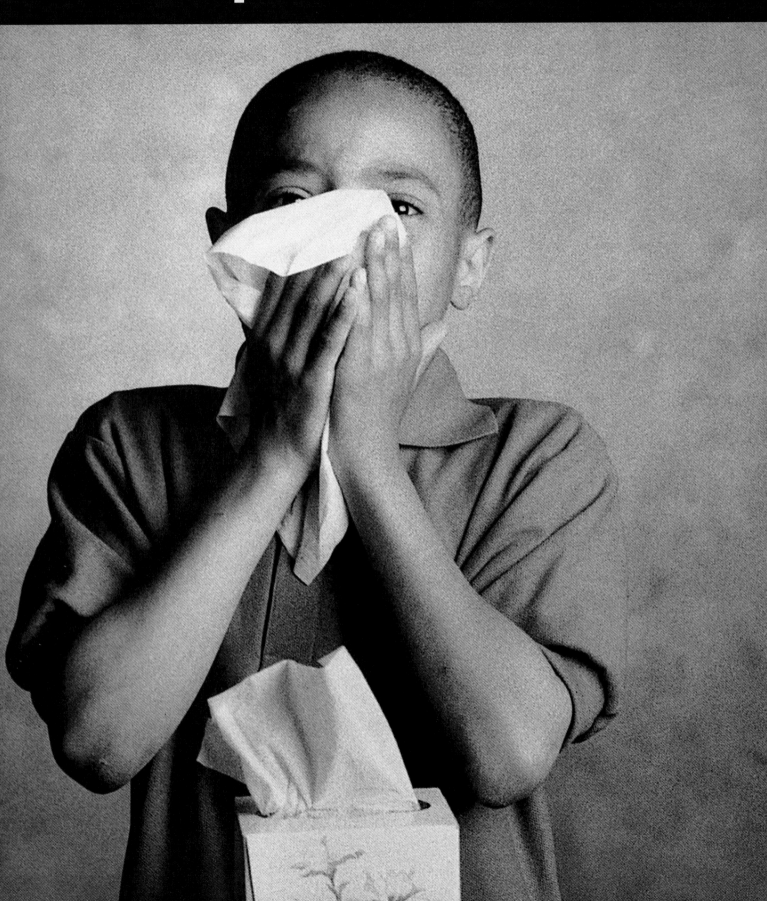

Communicable and Chronic Diseases

Lesson 25
Disease Defenders

Lesson 26
It's Catching

Lesson 27
Chronic Diseases

Lesson 28
What to Know About HIV and AIDS

Disease Defenders

Vocabulary

disease: an illness that keeps your body from working as it should.

bacteria: one-celled germs.

viruses: germs that are much smaller than bacteria.

body defenses: ways your body protects you from germs.

antibody: a substance in your blood that kills germs.

vaccine: a substance made with dead or weak germs.

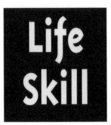

Life Skill

- I will choose habits that prevent the spread of germs.

You share toys with friends. You share good times with friends. These are good things to share. Some things are not good to share. You do not want to share germs with friends. Germs are tiny living things that can cause disease.

The Lesson Objectives

- Tell how germs cause disease.
- Name ways germs are spread.
- Tell ways to keep germs from entering your body.
- Tell ways to keep from spreading germs.
- Explain what body defenses do.

How Do Germs Cause Disease?

Disease is an illness that keeps your body from working as it should. Germs can cause disease. Bacteria and viruses are germs.

Bacteria cause diseases by making poisons.

Bacteria (bak·TIR·ee·uh) are one-celled germs. They have different shapes. They grow by splitting in two. Then the two split again into four, and so on.

Bacteria make poisons. The poisons cause infections and illness. Staph bacteria cause skin infections. Strep bacteria cause a throat infection. It is called strep throat.

Viruses cause disease by bursting cells.

Viruses (VY·ruh·suhz) are germs that are much smaller than bacteria. They have many different shapes. Viruses grow by making copies of themselves.

Viruses get inside your body cells. Then they make exact copies of themselves. Lots of the same virus is made within a cell. This causes cells to burst open. They die. The viruses then find other cells to get inside.

Viruses cause many diseases. Some of these are colds, flu, and chickenpox.

Drugs for Bacteria and Viruses

There are many drugs that kill bacteria. Antibiotics are one kind of drug. Antibiotics do not work against viruses.

There are only a few drugs that work against viruses. Some drugs keep viruses from making copies of themselves. Some drugs keep viruses from entering body cells.

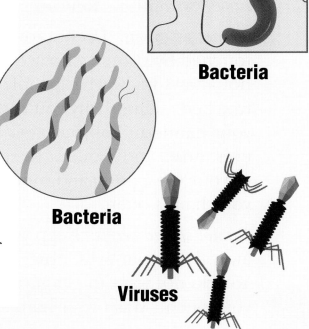

Bacteria

Bacteria

Viruses

How Are Germs Spread?

Germs are spread by breathing droplets from other people. You go into your sister's bedroom. She is in bed with the flu. She starts to sneeze. The droplets from a sneeze and cough contain germs. You might breathe the germs.

Do not get germs: Keep away from people who are sick.

Do not spread germs: Cover your nose and mouth when you cough or sneeze. Wash your hands afterwards.

Germs are spread by touching objects people have touched. A girl at school has a cold. She wipes her nose with her hand. Her germs get on her pencil. You borrow her pencil. The germs get on your hands. Suppose you put the pencil in your mouth. The germs can enter your body through your eyes, nose, or mouth. You can get sick.

Do not get germs: Do not touch objects touched by people who are sick. You do not always know what people have touched. This is why you should keep your hands and objects away from your eyes, nose, and mouth. Keep objects out of your eyes, nose, and mouth. Wash your hands often.

Do not spread germs: Keep your hands away from your eyes, nose, and mouth. You do not want to get germs on objects you touch. Wash your hands often.

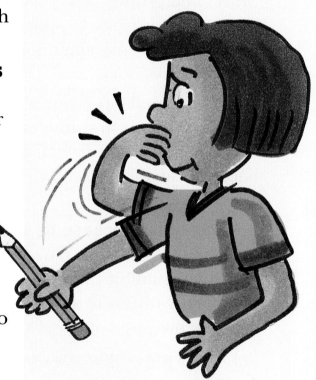

Germs can be spread from animals.

As you walk home from school, you see a strange dog. The dog looks friendly. You wonder if you should pet it.

Do not pet a strange dog. The dog could bite you. Germs can get in your body through the broken skin.

Do not get germs: Do not pet strange dogs. Keep mosquitoes and ticks off your body. Wear a special spray to keep them off your body.

Do not spread germs: Some germs you get from animals can be spread. Ask your doctor what to do if you get germs from an animal.

Germs are spread through food and water.

You go to a restaurant to eat. Your hamburger is bright pink in the middle. It is not cooked all the way through.

Do not eat the hamburger. Ask your server to have it cooked. Undercooked hamburger might contain germs. The germs can enter your body if you eat it. There are other foods that can contain germs.

Do not get germs: Do not eat undercooked hamburger and chicken. Do not leave food out that might spoil. Keep it in the refrigerator. Wash your hands before you touch food.

Do not spread germs: You can spread some germs you get from food to others. Always wash your hands after you use the bathroom. Do not prepare food for someone else when you are sick.

Soap and Scrub!

Many germs are spread by hands. Washing your hands is a very important action to fight germs. Wet your hands. Put soap on your hands. Rub your hands together while you count slowly to fifteen. Rub between your fingers and under your nails. Rinse and dry. Always wash your hands after you use the bathroom. Always wash your hands before you eat. Always wash your hands after you sneeze, cough, or blow your nose.

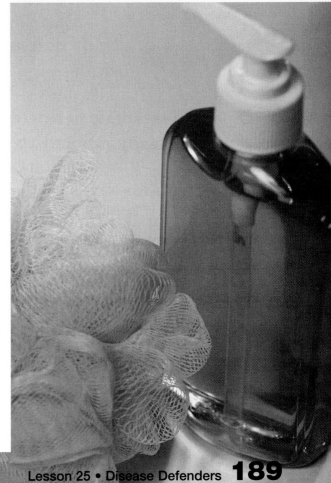

What Are My Body's Defenses?

Suppose you are at a football game. You hear people yell "defense." They want their team to defend their goal. To defend means to protect or guard. Each team tries to protect its goal. Your body defends you from germs. **Body defenses** are ways your body protects you from germs.

Your skin is a body defense. It defends you by keeping germs from entering your body. Germs can enter your body if your skin is cut or broken.

A white blood cell is a body defense. White blood cells defend you by destroying germs.

An antibody is a body defense. An **antibody** (AN·ti·bah·dee) is a substance in your blood that kills germs. Antibodies defend you by killing germs. Your body makes a different antibody to kill each kind of germ. Antibodies are made by your body in two ways.

- Your body makes antibodies each time you have a disease caused by a germ. The antibodies kill that kind of germ.

- Your body makes antibodies after you are given a vaccine. A **vaccine** (vak·SEEN) is a substance made with dead or weak germs. There are different kinds of vaccines. Each vaccine can protect you from a certain kind of germ.

Are You Up-to-Date on Vaccines?

By now, you should have had vaccines against these diseases: diphtheria (dif·THEER·ee·uh), tetanus (TET·uh·nuhs), pertussis (puhr·TUHS·is) (whooping cough), polio, measles, mumps, and rubella (roo·BEL·uh). If you have not had chickenpox, you should get the chickenpox vaccine.

Germ Fighters

Activity

Life Skill

- I will choose habits that prevent the spread of germs.

Materials: Peel-off labels, pen

Directions: This activity shows ways to prevent the spread of germs.

1. **Think of slogans that tell how to prevent the spread of germs.** A slogan is a message that is easy to remember. Examples are: "I drowned a germ" for someone who washes his hands; "The germ stops here" for someone who uses a tissue.

2. **Write your slogans on the peel-off labels.**

3. **Notice what your classmates do to prevent the spread of germs.**

4. **Give a sticker to each classmate who prevents the spread of germs.**

Lesson 25

Review

Vocabulary

Write a separate sentence using each vocabulary word listed on page 186.

Health Content

1. How do bacteria and viruses cause disease? **page 187**

2. What are ways germs are spread? **pages 188–189**

3. How can you keep from spreading germs? **pages 188–189**

4. How can you keep germs from entering your body? **pages 188–189**

5. What are some body defenses? **page 190**

It's Catching

Vocabulary

communicable disease: a disease that can be spread to people from people, animals, and the environment.

symptom: a change from normal in a person's health.

strep throat: a sore throat caused by a kind of bacteria.

infestation: having mites, ticks, lice, or worms.

head lice: tiny insects that lay eggs in the hair.

Life Skill

- **I will recognize symptoms and get treatment for communicable diseases.**

A **communicable** (kuh·MYOO·ni·kuh·buhl) **disease** is a disease that can be spread to people from people, animals, and the environment. You learned ways these diseases are spread in Lesson 25. You will learn ways to take care of yourself when you have a communicable disease.

The Lesson Objectives

- Discuss what to do if you have a cold or flu.
- Discuss what to do if you have a sore throat.
- Discuss how head lice are spread and treated.
- Discuss how scabies are spread and treated.
- Discuss how to keep from getting Lyme Disease.

What Should I Do If I Have a Cold, the Flu, or Strep Throat?

What to Do for a Cold or Flu

Colds and flu are caused by viruses. Symptoms are runny and stuffy nose, sneezing, coughing, and headache. A **symptom** is a change from normal in a person's health.

There is no cure for colds or flu. Get plenty of rest. Drink lots of fluids. Your doctor might tell your parent or guardian to give you an over-the-counter medicine. The medicine might lessen your coughing or sneezing.

Your parents or guardian might take you to a doctor if you have a bad cold or an earache. A doctor might want to see you if you have pain around your eyes. You could have another disease. Your doctor might give you antibiotics.

What to Do for a Sore Throat

A sore throat can be caused by bacteria or viruses. **Strep throat** is a sore throat caused by a kind of bacteria. Your doctor can tell you if you have strep throat. Your doctor might give you antibiotics. If not treated, strep throat can lead to heart and kidney disease.

There is no cure for a sore throat caused by viruses. Your doctor might tell your parent or guardian to give you an over-the-counter medicine.

Finish It Up!

You might have a sore throat or earache caused by bacteria. Your doctor might give you antibiotics. Take all the antibiotics. Do not stop when you feel better. All the bacteria might not be killed. They might grow. You might get another sore throat or earache.

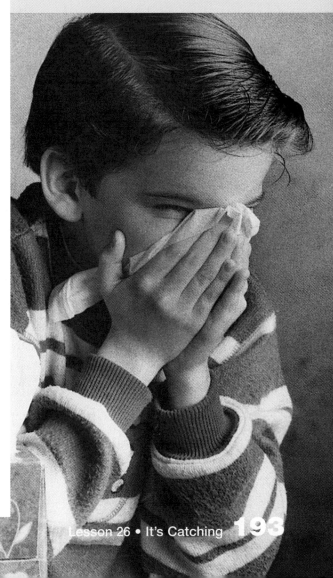

How Are Head Lice and Scabies Spread?

An **infestation** is having mites, ticks, lice, or worms. These animals are not germs. But they can be spread from person to person.

Head Lice

Head lice are tiny insects that lay eggs in the hair. They are about 1/8 inch long. Lice suck blood from your scalp. You itch where they suck blood. You might have sores and scabs where you scratch.

Head lice are spread by sharing hats, combs, and hairbrushes. You should not go to school with lice. Head lice are spread easily. Your parents or guardian can put a special shampoo on your scalp and hair. The shampoo kills the lice. Wash combs, hairbrushes, and hats in warm, soapy water.

Scabies

Scabies is a skin infestation caused by a mite. The mite burrows into your skin and lays eggs. The burrows can be seen as tiny, gray raised areas. You itch a lot if you have scabies. You might get sores and scabs from scratching.

You should not go to school with mites. The mites are spread easily. You can get mites from touching a person with mites. Your parents or guardian can put a special lotion on your body. The lotion kills the mites.

What Is Lyme Disease?

Ticks can carry bacteria that cause Lyme disease. Lyme disease can affect your brain and heart. The ticks live on deer. But the ticks can get on pets and on you!

Keep ticks off your body. Use an insect spray if you will be camping or hiking. Check your body for ticks often when you camp or hike through woods or grass. Tell an adult to remove ticks from you or a pet.

Symptoms of Lyme disease are tiredness, muscle pain, headache, and fever. Some people have a red rash that is several inches long. Antibiotics are used to treat Lyme disease.

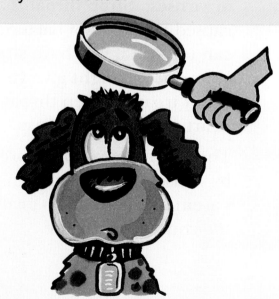

Use... Guidelines for Making Responsible Decisions™

Situation:

You and a friend are going camping. You take clothing to keep ticks off your body. You take an insect spray. Your friend says he is not worried about it. He tries to talk you into not protecting yourself.

Response:

Answer "yes" or "no" to each of the following questions. Explain each answer.

1. Is it healthful not to protect yourself?
2. Is it safe not to protect yourself?
3. Do you follow rules and laws if you do not protect yourself?
4. Do you show respect for yourself and others if you do not protect yourself?
5. Do you follow your family's guidelines if you do not protect yourself?
6. Do you show good character if you do not protect yourself?

What is the responsible decision to make?

Lesson 26

Review

Vocabulary

Write a separate sentence using each vocabulary word listed on page 192.

Health Content

1. What should you do if you have a cold or flu? **page 193**
2. What should you do if you have a sore throat? **page 193**
3. How are head lice spread and treated? **page 194**
4. How is scabies spread and treated? **page 194**
5. How can you keep from getting Lyme disease? **page 194**

Chronic Diseases

Vocabulary

chronic disease: a disease that lasts a long time.

heart disease: a disease of the heart and blood vessels.

cancer: a disease in which harmful cells grow.

allergy: the body's overreaction to a substance.

asthma: a condition in which the air passages become narrow.

Life Skills

- I will choose habits that prevent heart disease.
- I will choose habits that prevent cancer.
- I will tell ways to care for chronic (lasting) health conditions.
- I will tell ways to care for asthma and allergies.

A **chronic** (KRAH·nik) **disease** is a disease that lasts a long time. Heart disease and cancer are chronic diseases. Allergies and asthma also are chronic diseases.

The Lesson Objectives

- Name ways to keep from getting heart disease and cancer.
- Name things to which you can be allergic and ways you can lessen allergens from your pet.
- Name things that cause asthma attacks.

What Are Habits to Prevent Heart Disease and Cancer?

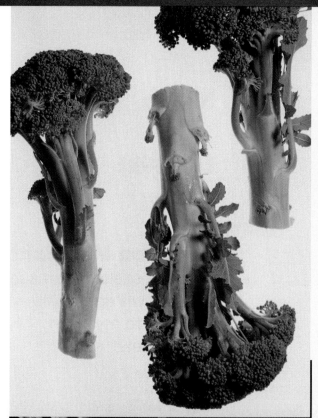

Heart disease is a disease of the heart and blood vessels. **Cancer** is a disease in which harmful cells grow.

Eat a healthful diet. Fatty foods can stick to your artery walls. This can block blood flow. Blood with oxygen in it might not reach your heart. This can cause a heart attack. A *heart attack* is a sudden loss of oxygen to the heart. Eat low-fat foods to prevent heart disease.

Eat low-fat foods to prevent cancer, too. Eat plenty of fiber. Fruits, vegetables, and grains have fiber in them. Fiber helps you have a daily bowel movement. This helps prevent cancer.

Keep away from tobacco. Nicotine in tobacco makes your heart beat faster. Your blood vessels get narrow. Then blood pressure must go up. This makes your heart work hard. Tobacco use causes heart disease.

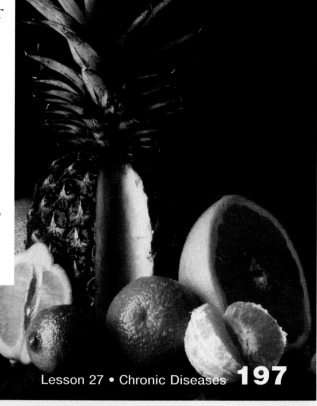

Tobacco use also causes cancer. Breathing smoke causes cancer, too. There are chemicals and harmful gases in smoke. There are harmful ingredients in smokeless tobacco. They cause cancer of the mouth, throat, and lungs.

Following the Health Behavior Contract

Name:_____ **Date:** _____

Life Skill: I will choose habits that prevent heart disease.

Effect on My Health: Heart disease is a disease of the heart and blood vessels. I can keep from getting heart disease when I am an adult. I will eat low-fat foods. My blood vessels will stay clear. Blood will flow to my heart. My heart will get the oxygen it needs. I will not have a heart attack.

My Plan: I will use the chart below. I will write the foods I eat for a week. I will put a check by the foods that are low-fat. I will ask my parent, guardian, or teacher to help me.

My Calendar	M	T	W	Th	F	S	S

How My Plan Worked: I put a check by the low-fat foods. I counted how many foods were low in fat.

What Can I Do If I Am Allergic to Pets?

An **allergy** (A·luhr·jee) is the body's overreaction to a substance. An *allergen* is a substance that causes the body to overreact.

You can have an allergy to something you breathe. You might be allergic to dust mites and pollen. *Dust mites* are tiny insects that live in carpets, mattresses, and dust. *Pollen* is a powdery substance in plants that can get in the air.

Any animal with fur and some birds can cause allergies. You are not allergic to the fur. You are allergic to an allergen in the saliva, dander, or urine. *Dander* is dead skin flakes.

You can lessen allergens from your pet.

Keep your pet outside your home as much as possible. Have a family member brush your pet outdoors. This will cut the amount of dander.

Keep your pet out of your bedroom. Do not let your pet in for even a short time. Allergens build up in mattresses, curtains, and carpets. They stay even after the pet has left. Vacuuming carpets does not help. It can stir up allergens.

Keep your pet and its living quarters clean. Have a family member clean the cage of rabbits, hamsters, and guinea pigs. Have this person give your pet a weekly bath. Ask your vet how to prevent dry skin on your pet.

Best Pet Bets

Dogs and cats cause most pet allergies. Cats cause worse reactions. What are the best pets if you are allergic? Any animal that does not have fur makes the best pet. Think about a turtle, hermit crab, or fish.

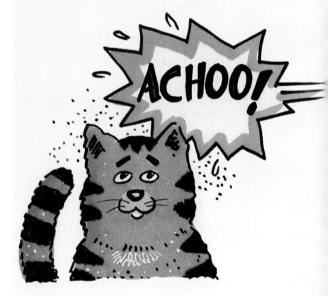

What Can Cause an Asthma Attack?

Asthma (AZ·muh) is a condition in which the air passages become narrow. This makes it hard to breathe in air. A person might have an asthma attack. During an asthma attack, a person might gasp. A person needs air.

Most of the time people who have asthma are OK. They have an asthma attack when they get around certain things. These things can cause people who have asthma to have an attack:

- **Pollen**
- **Animal dander**
- **Dust mites**

Someone in your class might have asthma. Many children have asthma. Children who have asthma might have an inhaler. An inhaler is a small device. It is used to spray medicine into the air passages. The medicine makes the air passages wider. Children who have asthma use the inhaler if breathing is hard. Then breathing gets easier.

Sometimes the medicine is not enough. A child might have to go to the hospital. A child might miss school for a few days.

Asthma is a condition in which the air passages become narrow.

Colds and Asthma

Colds and flu can make breathing hard for people who have asthma. If you have asthma, try not to get a cold or flu. Your parents or guardian might ask your doctor if you should get a flu shot. The best time to get a flu shot is between October 1 and November 15 every year. Keep away from other people who have colds or flu. Wash your hands with soap and water often. Keep your fingers out of your eyes, nose, and mouth. If you do not have asthma, be a friend to people who do. Do not spread your cold or flu to others. Cover your coughs and sneezes with a tissue. Wash your hands often.

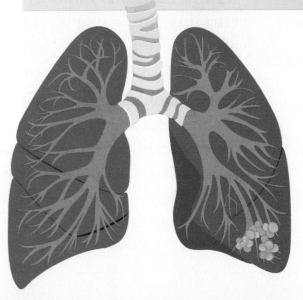

Use... Guidelines for Making Responsible Decisions™

Situation:

You are allergic to dander from cats. You have a hard time breathing near cats. You are in your friend's home. She has two cats. She says she will put the cats in another room.

Response:

Answer "yes" or "no" to each of the following questions. Explain each answer.

1. Is it healthful to go to the friend's home?

2. Is it safe to go to the friend's home?

3. Do you follow rules and laws if you go to the friend's home?

4. Do you show respect for yourself and others if you go to the friend's home?

5. Do you follow your family's guidelines if you go to the friend's home?

6. Do you show good character if you go to the friend's home?

What is the responsible decision to make?

Lesson 27

Review

Vocabulary

Write a separate sentence using each vocabulary word listed on page 196.

Health Content

1. What are habits to prevent heart disease and cancer? **page 197**

2. What are things to which you can be allergic? **page 199**

3. What can you do if you are allergic to pets? **page 199**

4. What can cause an asthma attack? **page 200**

5. What might happen if a child in your class has an asthma attack? **page 200**

What to Know About HIV and AIDS

Vocabulary

HIV: the germ that causes AIDS.

AIDS: an illness in which the body cannot fight diseases.

helper T cell: a special kind of white blood cell.

symptom: a change from normal in a person's health.

Life Skill

• I will learn facts about HIV and AIDS.

HIV is the germ that causes AIDS. **AIDS** is an illness in which the body cannot fight diseases. There is no cure for AIDS. This is why you need to know facts about HIV and AIDS. You can keep from getting AIDS.

The Lesson Objectives

• Explain what HIV does to helper T cells.

• Tell when a person has AIDS.

• Tell ways HIV is spread.

• Tell ways HIV is not spread.

• Tell ways to keep from getting HIV.

What Are Facts About HIV and AIDS?

A **helper T cell** is a special kind of white blood cell. Helper T cells help fight germs. A person stays well when the helper T cells work as they should.

HIV is the germ that causes AIDS. Suppose HIV gets into a person's blood. HIV attacks the helper T cells. It destroys some of them. Then there are fewer helper T cells.

A person who has HIV might not have symptoms right away. A **symptom** is a change from normal in a person's health. A person can look healthy. But HIV keeps destroying helper T cells. The number of helper T cells goes down. Sometimes it takes ten or more years for symptoms to show. Then a person who has HIV gets very tired. The person loses weight. The person has a fever. The person might have a hard time breathing.

A person has AIDS when the number of helper T cells is very low. There are not enough helper T cells to fight diseases.

I will learn facts about HIV and AIDS.

I will learn facts about HIV and AIDS.

I will learn facts about HIV and AIDS.

To date, there is no cure for AIDS. Scientists are working on a vaccine. They are working on treatments.

How Is HIV Spread?

HIV can be spread by touching blood that has HIV in it. Suppose a person who has HIV scrapes a knee. You press tissue on the knee to stop bleeding. The blood goes through the tissue. It gets into a tiny cut in your hand. HIV gets into your blood.

HIV can be spread by using a needle that has blood with HIV on it. Suppose a person who has HIV uses a needle to pierce ears. The person uses a needle to do harmful drugs. The needle has HIV on it. If you use the needle, HIV gets into your blood.

Ways HIV Is Not Spread

You cannot get HIV from a person who has HIV if you:

- sit next to the person.

- hug the person.

- shake hands with the person.

- use the same bathroom as the person.

- share a book or pencil with the person.

- breathe droplets from the person's coughs or sneezes.

How Can I Know If a Person Has HIV?

You cannot tell by looking at a person that he or she has HIV. People who have HIV can look and feel healthy. They might not even know they have HIV. The HIV can still be passed to you. Do not touch anyone's blood with your bare hands. Do not share needles with anyone. This includes people you know.

How Can I Keep from Getting HIV?

Do not touch someone else's blood.
Wear throw-away gloves if you help someone who is bleeding. Wash your hands with soap and water afterwards.

Do not press your cut finger against the finger of another person. This is sometimes done to become a blood brother or sister.

Do not share a needle. Suppose you share a needle to pierce ears or a body part. The needle can have blood on it. Never pierce ears or body parts without permission. A sterile needle must be used. Suppose you use a needle to put harmful drugs in your body. The needle can have blood on it. Do not use harmful drugs.

I will learn facts about HIV and AIDS.

I will learn facts about HIV and AIDS.

I will learn facts about HIV and AIDS.

Lesson 28

Review

Vocabulary

Write a separate sentence using each vocabulary word listed on page 202.

Health Content

1. What does HIV do to helper T cells?
   page 203
2. When does a person have AIDS?
   page 203
3. What are ways HIV is spread?
   page 204
4. What are ways HIV is not spread?
   page 204
5. What are ways to keep from getting HIV? **page 205**

Unit 7 Review

Health Content

1. How do bacteria cause disease? **Lesson 25 page 187**

2. What are two ways your body makes antibodies? **Lesson 25 page 190**

3. What are three things you can do when you have a cold? **Lesson 26 page 193**

4. How can a person get scabies? **Lesson 26 page 194**

5. What are ways to keep ticks off your body? **Lesson 26 page 194**

6. What are habits that keep you from getting heart disease? **Lesson 27 page 197**

7. How can you lessen allergens from pets? **Lesson 27 page 199**

8. What can happen when a person who has asthma breathes certain things? **Lesson 27 page 200**

9. How can HIV enter the body? **Lesson 28 page 204**

10. How can you NOT get HIV? **Lesson 28 page 204**

Guidelines for Making Responsible Decisions™

You are at the movies with a friend. You and your friend go to the restroom. Your friend does not wash her hands. She tells you it is not important. Answer "yes" or "no" to each of the following questions. Explain each answer.

1. Is it healthful not to wash your hands after you use the restroom?

2. Is it safe not to wash your hands after you use the restroom?

3. Do you follow rules and laws if you do not wash your hands after you use the restroom?

4. Do you show respect for yourself and others if you do not wash your hands after you use the restroom?

5. Do you follow your family's guidelines if you do not wash your hands after you use the restroom?

6. Do you show good character if you do not wash your hands after you use the restroom?

What is the responsible decision to make?

Vocabulary

Number a sheet of paper from 1–10. Read each definition. Next to each number on your sheet of paper, write the vocabulary word that matches the definition.

AIDS	heart disease
allergy	helper T cell
body defenses	infestation
chronic disease	strep throat
disease	vaccine

1. The body's overreaction to a substance. **Lesson 27**
2. Having mites, ticks, lice, or worms. **Lesson 26**
3. An illness in which the body cannot fight diseases. **Lesson 28**
4. Ways your body protects you from germs. **Lesson 25**
5. A disease of the heart and blood vessels. **Lesson 27**
6. A sore throat caused by a kind of bacteria. **Lesson 26**
7. A special kind of white blood cell. **Lesson 28**
8. A disease that lasts a long time. **Lesson 27**
9. An illness that keeps your body from working as it should. **Lesson 25**
10. A substance made with dead or weak germs. **Lesson 25**

Health Literacy

Effective Communication

Pretend a friend has a cold. What would you tell your friend to do to get better?

Self-Directed Learning

Look in an encyclopedia. Look up a disease to which you have been vaccinated. Write three facts about that disease.

Critical Thinking

Being a blood brother or blood sister means you are very close friends. What is a way to become a blood brother or blood sister without sharing blood?

Responsible Citizenship

Make a poster. Write three ways a person can keep from spreading germs. Put the poster where other people can see it.

Family Involvement

Go with your parents or guardian to the grocery store. Buy and try a fruit or vegetable your family has never eaten.

Unit 8

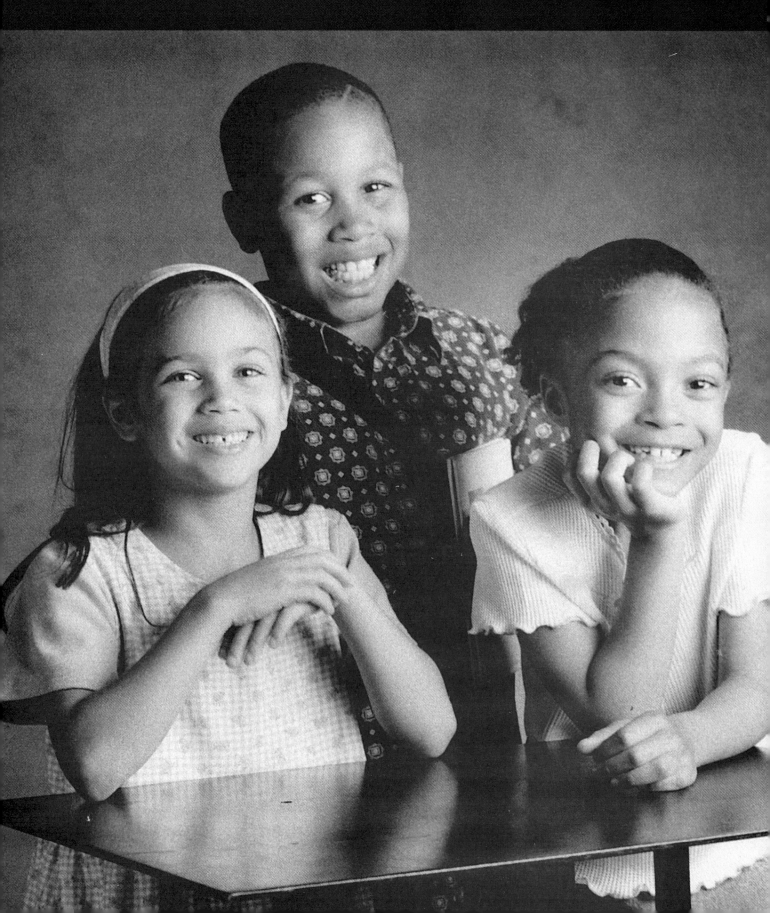

Consumer and Community Health

Check Out the Facts

Vocabulary

health information: facts about health.

health helper: a person who helps you stay healthy.

reliable information: information that is based on scientific study.

World Wide Web (Web): a computer system that lets a person find information, pictures, and text.

advertisement: a paid announcement.

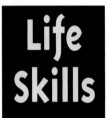

Life Skills

- I will check out sources of health information.
- I will check ways technology, media, and culture influence health choices.
- I will choose safe and healthful products.

Do you check out facts about health? Do you ask questions about a product before you buy it? Do you look for information about ways to be healthy? Checking out health information can help you make safe and healthful decisions.

The Lesson Objectives

- Explain when you are a consumer.
- Describe ways you can get health information.
- Tell how you can check out commercials for health products.

When Am I a Consumer?

You are a consumer when you check out health information. Health information is facts about health. You can learn ways to stay healthy. You can learn about diseases and problems.

You are a consumer when you buy health products. Suppose you go to a store with your parent or guardian. You ask your parent or guardian to buy you a new kind of toothpaste. Toothpaste is a health product. You are a consumer when you decide which toothpaste to buy.

You are a consumer when you use health services. Suppose you go to the doctor. The doctor provides a health service. The doctor helps you stay healthy. As a consumer, you can ask questions about the health service. For example, the doctor might want to give you a test. You can ask what the test will tell the doctor.

You are a consumer when you decide how to spend time and money. There are many ways you can spend your time and money.

You are a consumer when you choose entertainment. *Entertainment* (EN·tuhr·TAYN·muhnt) is something that interests or amuses you. You need to choose healthful entertainment.

A *consumer* is a person who:

- checks out health information.
- buys health products.
- uses health services.
- decides how to spend time and money.
- chooses entertainment.

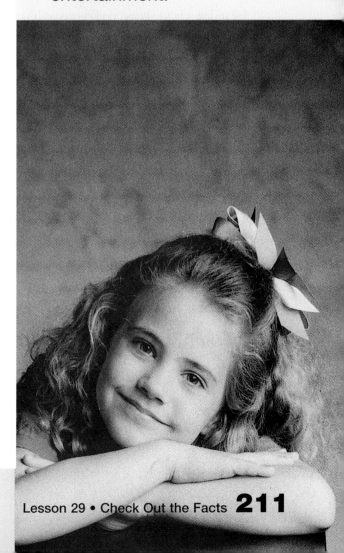

What Are Ways I Can Get Health Information?

You learn health information from this textbook. You learn health information from your teacher and your parents or guardian. There are many other ways you can learn health information.

Use the library. Your library has books about health. You can read about nutrition, how your body works, diseases, physical activity, and much more. Your library has encyclopedias. An *encyclopedia* (in·SY·kluh·PEE·dee·uh) is a set of books that has information on many subjects. Encyclopedias have articles on health. Your library might have magazines about health. These magazines have new health information. Ask a librarian to help you find information.

Take classes. Your health class teaches you about health. The American Red Cross gives classes in first aid. Local hospitals often give classes on health.

Ask a health helper. A **health helper** is a person who helps you stay healthy. A doctor is a health helper. A nurse is a health helper. You can ask these health helpers when you have questions about health.

Make Sure Health Information Is Reliable

Reliable (re·LY·uh·buhl) **information** is information that is based on scientific study. Reliable information comes from well-known health groups. It comes from doctors and scientists. It does not try to get you to buy anything. Other health groups and doctors believe reliable information. You must be very careful when you get health information from the World Wide Web. Anyone can put information on the Web. Make sure your health information on the Web comes from a well-known health group.

Use computer programs and games.

You can get computer programs and games to help you learn about health. These programs and games might come on a CD-ROM. A *CD-ROM* (SEE·DEE·RAHM) is a computer disc that stores computer programs. Programs and games on CD-ROMs can include words, pictures, music, speech, and movies. You might get information from an encyclopedia on a CD-ROM.

Use the World Wide Web.

The **World Wide Web,** or Web, is a computer system that lets a person find information, pictures, and text. A *Web site* is information put on the Web by a certain group. Get permission from a parent or guardian before you use the Web.

Many health services put information on the Web. Government groups that deal with health put information on the Web. The American Cancer Society and the American Heart Association are two groups that put health information on the Web. Many health groups have special information just for young people. They might include games and stories.

Check out a computer newsgroup.

A *newsgroup* is a place on a computer system where people can write questions and read answers. Ask a parent or guardian to help you if you want to look for information in a newsgroup. There are newsgroups for people who have certain diseases, such as diabetes.

Safety on the Web

- Get permission before you use the World Wide Web. Tell your parents or guardian what information you want. Tell them what Web sites you plan to look at. Look only at Web sites that are approved for children your age.

- Do not give personal information to anyone on a computer system.

- Do not use your last name if you write a question to a newsgroup.

- Do not give your address, telephone number, or any other information to anyone on a computer system.

- Tell your parents or guardian right away if you see any scary messages, pictures, or other information. Tell them if anyone tries to find out where you live.

How Can I Protect My Health When I Use a Computer?

Use correct posture. Sit up straight with your feet flat on the floor. Rest your feet on something if you cannot reach the floor while you sit in your chair. Place your keyboard and mouse low enough that you do not have to reach up to use them. You should be able to look straight ahead at your screen, not up or down. This will protect your neck, back, and arms.

Warm up muscles in your wrists and fingers. Run your hands and wrists under warm water for a few minutes before you use the computer. This warms up your muscles and helps blood flow. You are less likely to injure your muscles if you warm them up before you use the computer.

Keep your wrists flat while you type. Move your whole arm when you type or move the mouse. Rest your wrists on a wrist rest when you are not typing or using the mouse. Type lightly. Do not pound the keys.

Rest your eyes. Look away from the screen for a minute every 15 to 20 minutes. Look at something out the window or across the room. This rests your eyes. Your eyes can get tired if you stare at a computer screen for a long time.

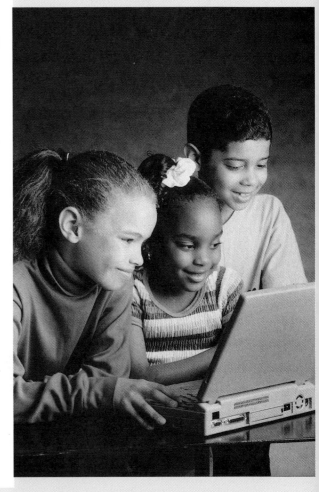

Find a Reference Book

Life Skill

● I will check out sources of health information.

Materials: Paper, pencil

Directions: You need to know how to find health information in the library. Follow the directions below to learn how to find a health reference.

Activity

1. **Use your school library.** Look up "first aid" in the card catalog or on the computer system.

2. **Write down the names of two books on first aid.** Write down the authors' names. Write down the call number that tells you where to find the books. A call number is a number that tells you where the book is in the library.

3. **Find the two books.** Find the row that has the call number for each book.

4. **Find the health information you want in the two books.** Look at the table of contents or the index in each book. Find the page that tells first aid for choking. Look at the page. Write down the page number of the section on choking next to the name of each book.

How Can I Check Out Commercials for Health Products?

An **advertisement** (AD·vuhr·TYZ·muhnt), or ad, is a paid announcement. Companies who make health products pay people to make ads. The ads are put in magazines for you to see. They are put on billboards for you to hear. A *commercial* (kuh·MUHR·shuhl) is an ad on radio or television.

Much money is spent on commercials. People who make commercials want you to buy something. They put music you will like in their commercials. They put famous people in them. They choose colors you like. The commercial might say a product will make others like you. It might say you will have more fun.

You can be a wise consumer. You can look for facts in commercials. You can check to see if facts are left out. Suppose there is a commercial for potato chips. It leaves out facts about how much fat is in them.

You can understand why you like a TV commercial. You can watch one without having to buy something. You can see if a product is healthful for you.

Use Questions to Check Out Commercials

- What product is in the commercial?
- What are ways the commercial tries to get me to want the product?
- What facts about the product are in the commercial?
- What facts about the product are left out of the commercial?
- Do I need the product?

Use... Guidelines for Making Responsible Decisions™

Situation:

You see an ad for a breakfast cereal. You really like the ad. The cereal is coated with sugar.

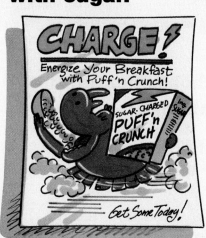

Response:

Answer "yes" or "no" to each of the following questions. Explain each answer.

1. Is it healthful to buy sugar-coated cereal because you like the ad?

2. Is it safe to buy sugar-coated cereal because you like the ad?

3. Do you follow rules and laws if you buy sugar-coated cereal because you like the ad?

4. Do you show respect for yourself and others if you buy sugar-coated cereal because you like the ad?

5. Do you follow your family's guidelines if you buy sugar-coated cereal because you like the ad?

6. Do you show good character if you buy sugar-coated cereal because you like the ad?

What is the responsible decision to make?

Lesson 29

Review

Vocabulary

Write a separate sentence using each vocabulary word listed on page 210.

Health Content

1. When are you a consumer? **page 211**

2. What are ways you can get health information? **pages 212–213**

3. How can you stay safe when you use the World Wide Web? **page 213**

4. How do you find a health book at a library? **page 215**

5. How can you check out commercials for health products? **page 216**

Entertainment Choices

Vocabulary

entertainment: something that interests or amuses you.

healthful entertainment: entertainment that promotes health.

hobby: something you like to do in your spare time.

organized: to keep track of your time and your belongings.

allowance: an amount of money your parents or guardian give you to spend.

Life Skills

- I will choose healthful entertainment.
- I will spend time and money wisely.

You spend time each day sleeping, eating, caring for yourself, and going to school. You choose what you will do for several hours each day. How do you spend your time? Do you plan your time to include homework and other activities? Do you choose healthful activities?

The Lesson Objectives

- Discuss kinds of healthful entertainment.
- Explain how you can stay organized.
- List questions to answer to check out TV shows.

What Are Kinds of Healthful Entertainment?

Entertainment (EN·tuhr·TAYN·muhnt) is something that interests or amuses you. **Healthful entertainment** is entertainment that promotes health.

Physical activity is healthful entertainment. You can have fun and keep your body healthy. You can meet people who enjoy the same activities you enjoy. You might enjoy in-line skating with a friend.

Hobbies are healthful entertainment. A **hobby** is something you like to do in your spare time. You might enjoy collecting something, building model airplanes, doing art projects, or playing the piano. You learn to do something well when you practice a hobby. You can meet people who have the same hobby.

Reading is healthful entertainment. You become a better reader and learn new words. You can do better in school when you read for fun.

Being in a club is healthful entertainment. You can join a club of people who enjoy the things you enjoy. You can learn crafts, go camping, and make new friends in clubs.

Some TV shows and movies are healthful entertainment. They show families solving problems in healthful ways. They show people choosing healthful behavior.

Clubs You Might Join

Boy Scouts or Girl Scouts

Boys and Girls Clubs

4-H

Campfire Boys and Girls

Local sports groups

Local hobby groups

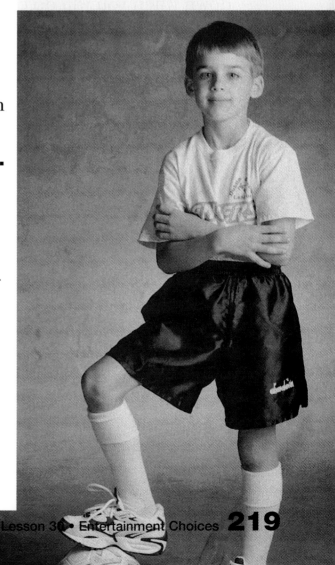

How Can I Stay Organized?

To be **organized** (OR·guh·NYZD) is to keep track of your time and your belongings. You can plan activities to make sure you do everything you want to do in a day.

Know what you must do in a day. Try this for one day. Write down what time you will get up and what time you will go to bed. Write down when you will bathe and eat. Write down the hours you will spend in school. Write down when you will do chores and homework. Plan time for family members and time to be alone. Plan healthful entertainment.

Stick to your plan for getting things done. Follow your plan for one day. Were you able to do everything you planned? You do not have to plan every minute of every day. You should plan to do some things, like homework, at the same time every day.

Keep your belongings in order. This helps save time. Keep your room clean and neat. Keep your desk at school clean and neat. You will be able to find things easily. Keep your tests and homework papers neat. You might put them in a folder or notebook. Keep your clothing neatly folded or hung up. You will not waste time looking for clothes.

Manage Your Money

You might get an allowance. An **allowance** (uh·LOW·uhnts) is an amount of money your parents or guardian give you to spend. You might earn money for chores. You should save part of any money you get. Suppose you want to buy something. Ask yourself these questions:

- Do I need this item?
- Do I need it right now?
- What will happen if I do not have this item?

Do not buy the item if you answer "no" to either of the first two questions. Do not buy the item if you answer that "nothing will happen" or "it will not matter" to the third question.

Checking Out TV Shows

Life Skill

- I will choose healthful entertainment.

Materials: Permission to watch a TV program, paper, pencil

Directions: Check out your favorite TV show. Watch the show. Write answers to the questions below.

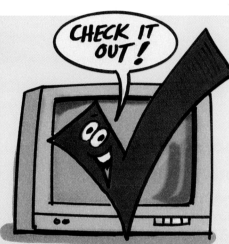

CHECK IT OUT!

How to Check Out a TV Show

- Does the TV show tell me to follow family guidelines?
- Do the people in the TV show act in responsible ways?
- Does the TV show leave out violence?
- Does the TV show leave out bad words?
- Do I have permission from my parents or guardian to watch this TV show?

Lesson 30

Review

Vocabulary

Write a separate sentence using each vocabulary word listed on page 218.

Health Content

1. What are five kinds of healthful entertainment? **page 219**

2. What are reasons to have a hobby? **page 219**

3. What are reasons to read for entertainment? **page 219**

4. How can you stay organized? **page 220**

5. What are questions to ask to check out TV shows? **page 220**

Health Helpers

Vocabulary

health helper: a person who helps you stay healthy.

doctor: a person who is trained to treat people who are ill or injured.

nurse: a person who is trained to take care of sick or injured people and who is supervised by a doctor.

police officer: a person who keeps you safe by making sure people follow laws.

Life Skills

- I will cooperate with community and school health helpers.
- I will learn about health careers.

There are many people who work to help you stay healthy. These people are called health helpers. A **health helper** is a person who helps you stay healthy. You know that a doctor or a nurse is a health helper. Did you know that your teacher is a health helper? Police and firefighters are health helpers, too.

The Lesson Objectives

- Tell what health helpers in your school do.
- Tell what health helpers at the doctor's office and hospital do.
- Tell what health helpers in your community do.

Who Are Health Helpers in My School?

Your teacher is a health helper.
Your teacher helps you learn life skills. A *life skill* is a healthful action you learn and practice for life. Your teacher helps protect your health and safety. Your teacher gets the school nurse if you are ill or injured. Your teacher tells you what to do if there is a fire or storm.

Your physical education teacher is a health helper. He or she teaches you how to play sports and games. This teacher helps you get ready to take a physical fitness test.

The school nurse is a health helper. The *school nurse* takes care of students who get sick or hurt at school. The school nurse helps take care of students who have chronic diseases. A classmate might have medicine to take. The school nurse keeps the medicine. The school nurse gives your classmate the medicine at the right times. The school nurse might come into your class and teach about health.

A dietitian is a health helper. A *dietitian* (DY·uh·TI·shuhn) is a person who plans healthful meals and runs a kitchen. Your school might have a dietitian. The dietitian plans school lunches to make sure they are healthful. The dietitian might buy food and cooking supplies. He or she might run the school kitchen.

Learn About School Health Helpers

Do you think you might like to be a school health helper when you grow up? Ask the health helpers at your school about their jobs. Check out books at the library about each job. You can learn what classes you will need to take when you get older.

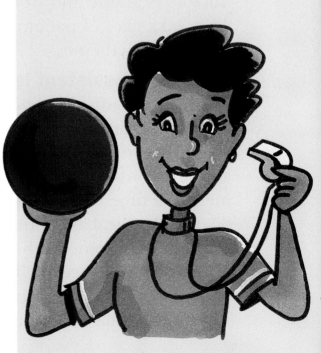

Who Are Health Helpers at the Doctor's Office and Hospital?

You see many different people when you go to a doctor's office or hospital. They all work together to help keep you healthy.

A doctor is a health helper. A **doctor** is a person who is trained to treat people who are ill or injured. A doctor examines you when you go to a doctor's office or hospital. The doctor might order tests to find out about your health. The doctor might prescribe medicine to make you well.

A nurse is a health helper. A **nurse** is a person who is trained to take care of sick or injured people and who is supervised by a doctor. Nurses help doctors examine and treat patients. They take care of patients in hospitals. They give medicines.

A medical assistant is a health helper. A *medical assistant* is a person who helps run a doctor's office. Medical assistants answer telephones and make appointments for patients. An appointment is a time when you can see the doctor. Medical assistants check patients in when they come to the office. They check patients' record. They weigh patients and ask about their health. They might take blood or urine for tests.

Ask Questions

Suppose you go to the doctor's office. The doctor wants to do a test. You do not understand the test. Ask! Your doctor can explain why the test is needed. Your doctor can explain what will happen during the test. You will feel better if you understand what is happening.

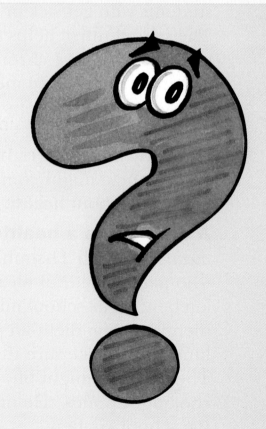

A pharmacist is a health helper.

A *pharmacist* (FAR·muh·sist) is a person who gives out medicine your doctor prescribes. Pharmacists work in pharmacies. A *pharmacy* (FAR·muh·see) is a place where prescription drugs are given out or sold. There are pharmacies in hospitals, grocery stores, drug stores, and other places.

Pharmacists make sure you get the right number of pills. They tell you the correct way to take drugs. For example, you might need to take a medicine with food. Pharmacists tell you about side effects. A *side effect* is an unwanted feeling or illness after taking a medicine. Pharmacists also tell doctors which drugs help certain diseases. They tell doctors if two drugs should not be taken at the same time.

A dietitian is a health helper.

Some dietitians work in hospitals. They do some of the same things they do in schools. They also decide what foods are best for people who have certain diseases. They help people who have certain diseases plan meals to eat at home.

A medical record technician is a health helper.

A *medical record technician* (TEC·ni·shuhn) is a person who makes sure your health records are clear. When your doctor examines you, he or she writes information on a chart. When you have a test or an operation, the doctor writes it down. Medical record technicians keep charts and other records in order.

When a Loved One Is in the Hospital

Suppose a family member is in the hospital. You might be able to visit the family member. Tell your family member you love him or her. You might make a get-well card for your family member.

A hospital rule might say that children your age cannot visit in the hospital. You can still make a card and ask an adult to give it to the family member. You can ask the adult to tell the family member you are thinking of him or her.

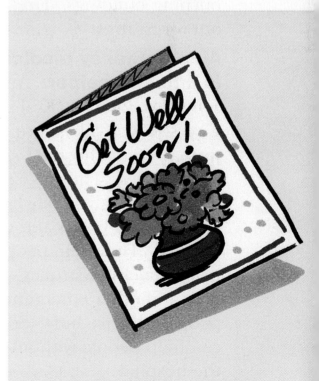

Who Are Health Helpers in the Community?

A police officer is a health helper.
A **police officer** is a person who keeps
you safe by making sure people follow
laws. Police officers check your neighborhood to make sure nothing is wrong.
They arrest people who are violent or
who harm others. They can help you if
you are lost or hurt.

A firefighter is a health helper. A
firefighter is a person who puts out fires
and helps people in emergencies.
Firefighters help people who have been
in car accidents. They help people
during earthquakes and floods. They
rescue people who are trapped inside
burning buildings. Firefighters also put
out forest fires.

**An emergency medical technician
is a health helper.** An *emergency medical technician* (TECK·ni·shuhn) *(EMT)* is
a person who takes care of people on
the way to the hospital. EMTs drive
ambulances. They take people to the
hospital quickly. They help people who
have broken bones and other major
injuries. They help people who have
heart attacks or strokes. EMTs go to
fires and other emergencies to help
people who are hurt. Sometimes, EMTs
can help people without taking them to
the hospital.

Health Helper for Your Pet

Pets need health care,
too. A *veterinarian*
(VE·tuh·ruh·NEHR·ee·uhn)
is a doctor who takes
care of animals. Perhaps
you have taken a pet to
the veterinarian. The
veterinarian examined
your pet. Your pet might
have needed shots. Your
pet might have needed
a test or some medicine.
Veterinarians must know
about many kinds of
animals. They must
know what medicines
work for each animal.

Health Helper Thank-You Card

Life Skill

- I will cooperate with community and school health helpers.

Materials: Construction paper, markers, pencil

Directions: Follow the directions below to make a thank-you card for a health helper.

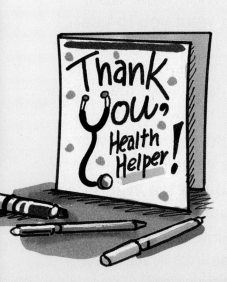

1. **Make a thank-you card using the construction paper.** Choose a health helper who helps you or someone in your family. Write "Thank You, Health Helper" on the front of the card. Decorate the front of the card.

2. **Write a note to the health helper on the inside of the card.** Your note should include how the health helper has helped you and why you are glad the health helper is there.

3. **Sign your name inside the card.** Give your card to your health helper.

Activity

Lesson 31

Review

Vocabulary

Write a separate sentence using each vocabulary word listed on page 222.

Health Content

1. Who are health helpers in your school? **page 223**

2. Who are health helpers at the doctor's office and hospital? **pages 224–225**

3. What does a pharmacist do? **page 225**

4. Who are health helpers in your community? **page 226**

5. What does a veterinarian do? **page 226**

Unit 8 Review

Health Content

1. What are ways you are a consumer? **Lesson 29 page 211**

2. How can you protect your health when you use a computer? **Lesson 29 page 214**

3. What are questions you can ask yourself when you see a commercial? **Lesson 29 page 216**

4. What are five kinds of healthful entertainment you might choose? **Lesson 30 page 219**

5. What are three ways you can stay organized? **Lesson 30 page 220**

6. What questions can you ask to check out a TV show? **Lesson 30 page 221**

7. What do health helpers in your school do? **Lesson 31 page 223**

8. How can you learn about school health helpers? **Lesson 31 page 223**

9. What do health helpers in a doctor's office and hospital do? **Lesson 31 pages 224–225**

10. Who are three health helpers in the community? **Lesson 31 page 226**

Guidelines for Making Responsible Decisions™

You are at a friend's house. Your friend suggests that the two of you use the World Wide Web. Your parents do not want you to use the World Wide Web without their permission. Answer "yes" or "no" to each of the following questions. Explain each answer.

1. Is it healthful to use the World Wide Web without permission?

2. Is it safe to use the World Wide Web without permission?

3. Do you follow rules and laws if you use the World Wide Web without permission?

4. Do you show respect for yourself and others if you use the World Wide Web without permission?

5. Do you follow your family's guidelines if you use the World Wide Web without permission?

6. Do you show good character if you use the World Wide Web without permission?

What is the responsible decision to make?

Vocabulary

Number a sheet of paper from 1–10. Read each definition. Next to each number on your sheet of paper, write the vocabulary word that matches the definition.

health helper	advertisement
allowance	health information
organized	hobby
entertainment	police officer
reliable information	doctor

1. A person who is trained to treat people who are ill or injured. **Lesson 31**
2. An amount of money your parents or guardian give you to spend. **Lesson 30**
3. Something that interests or amuses you. **Lesson 30**
4. Something you like to do in your spare time. **Lesson 30**
5. To keep track of your time and your belongings. **Lesson 30**
6. A person who keeps you safe by making sure people follow laws. **Lesson 31**
7. A paid announcement. **Lesson 29**
8. Information that is based on scientific study. **Lesson 29**
9. A person who helps you stay healthy. **Lesson 31**
10. Facts about health. **Lesson 29**

Health Literacy

Effective Communication

Make a poster that shows the correct way to use a computer. Write ways to protect your wrists, neck, back, arms, fingers, and eyes.

Self-Directed Learning

Use the library. Find a book about a hobby that interests you. Try out the hobby.

Critical Thinking

Answer the following question on a sheet of paper. Why is it important to tell your parents or guardian if you see any scary pictures or text on the World Wide Web?

Responsible Citizenship

Get permission from your parents or guardian to ask a health helper five questions about his or her job.

Family Involvement

Watch a TV show with your parents or guardian. Ask the questions on page 216 about two commercials you see during the show. Discuss your answers.

Unit 9

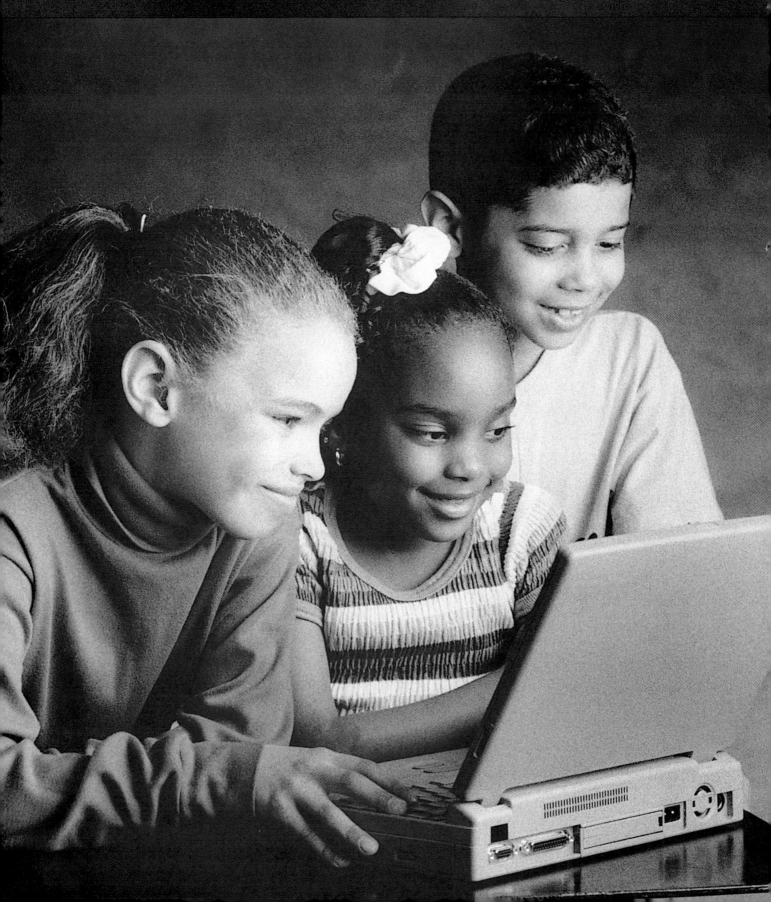

Environmental Health

Clean-Up Crew

Vocabulary

environment:
everything that
is around you.

pollution:
substances in the
environment that
can harm health.

litter: trash that
is thrown on land
or in water.

water pollution:
substances in water
that make it unclean
and harmful.

air pollution:
substances in the
air that make it
unsafe to breathe.

Life Skills

- I will help protect
  my environment.
- I will keep the air, land,
  and water clean and safe.

Your **environment** (in·VY·ruhn·muhnt)
is everything that is around you. Your
community is the place where the people
around you live. A clean-up crew is a group
of people who keep your community clean.
Everyone in your community must be part of
the clean-up crew.

The Lesson Objectives

- Discuss ways your community is
  kept clean.
- Discuss kinds of pollution.
- Tell ways to keep your community clean.

How Is My Community Kept Clean?

Your community might have garbage service. *Garbage* is food and other things that are thrown out. You might put garbage in bags. Then you might put the bags in a container at your apartment.

Your family might put the garbage bags by the street. This is done on a certain day of the week. People who collect garbage come that day. They collect the bags and throw them in a truck. The truck takes the garbage to a landfill. A *landfill* is a place where waste is dumped and buried.

Your community has treatment plants to make water clean and safe. Suppose you flush water down the toilet. Suppose you pour water down the drain. This water will be used again. But first it must be cleaned. A *waste-treatment plant* is a place where water is cleaned. A *water-treatment plant* is a place where water is treated and made safe to drink.

Your community might have volunteers who help keep it clean. A *volunteer* is someone who works without pay. Some volunteers might pick up trash in a park. Other volunteers take care of other places in your community.

The Adopt-a-Highway Program

The *Adopt-a-Highway Program* is a program in which volunteers pick up trash to keep highways clean. Volunteers must be 12 years old or older. They wear orange safety vests so drivers can see them.

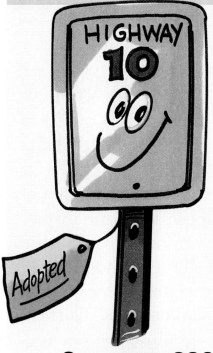

See page 236 for ways you can keep your community clean.

What Are Kinds of Pollution?

Pollution (puh·LOO·shuhn) is substances in the environment that can harm health. There are different kinds of pollution.

Litter is pollution Litter is trash that is thrown on land or in water. Paper, metal cans, plastic, and glass can be litter. Litter can be food. Suppose someone throws a soda can out the window of a car. Suppose someone leaves paper from fast food on the street. It is against the law to throw litter in a public place.

Litter can cause you and others to get sick. Suppose food is on your street. Flies and other insects come to where the food is. Wild animals come to where the food is. They carry germs. You are more likely to get sick. Places where there is litter are dirty.

Litter can be unsafe for you and others. Suppose someone throws a bottle out a car window. It lands on the playground and shatters into pieces. You and your friends play there. Someone might step on broken glass. Germs on the broken glass get into the person's body. The person gets an infection.

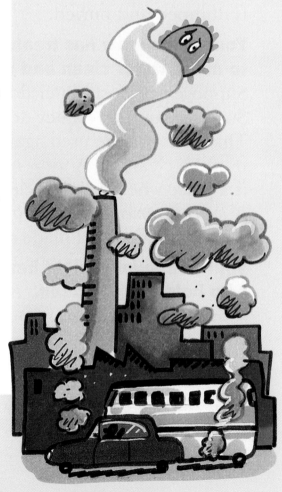

Water pollution Water pollution is substances in water that make it unclean and harmful. Litter is one cause of water pollution. People might throw garbage in water.

Some people who work at factories pollute water. They dump wastes from their factory into a nearby river, lake, or stream. Some farmers pollute water. They put chemicals on their crops. These chemicals end up on the ground. When it rains, the rain water flows to a nearby river, lake, or stream. The rain water has the chemicals in it. Some people dump chemicals into the water.

Suppose a woman changes the oil in her car. She might pour it down a drain. She might pour it on the ground. It gets into the water supply.

Polluted water is unsafe to drink. Chemicals in the water can be unsafe. Germs can be in polluted water. Suppose animals or fish live in polluted water. They are unsafe to eat. Suppose plants are watered with polluted water. They are unsafe to eat.

Air pollution Air pollution is substances in the air that make it unsafe to breathe. Waste from cars and smoke from buildings are a cause. Secondhand smoke is a cause. Suppose you breathe polluted air. You might cough. Your heart rate can go up. You might have more respiratory infections. You can get lung cancer.

What If I Eat Fish from Polluted Water?

You can get sick if you eat fish that were in polluted water. They can have chemicals in them. They can have germs in them.

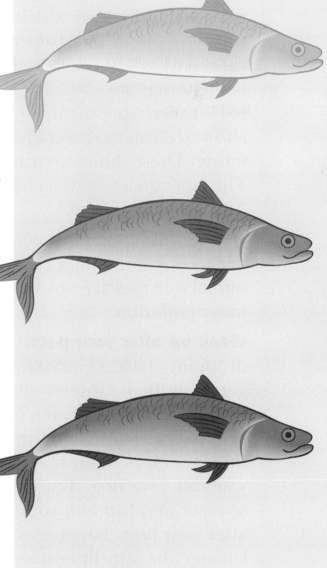

How Can I Keep My Community Clean?

Do not litter. Do not throw papers from fast foods on the ground. Do not toss things out your car window. Always put trash in a trash can.

Do not pollute water. Be careful what you pour down the drain. Be careful what you flush down a toilet. Be careful what you put in a garbage disposal. Be careful what you pour on the ground. Some things are safe. They are: water, toilet paper, soap, shampoo, some sink and tub cleaners, beverages, and food waste. These things are carried in water. The water goes to a waste treatment plant. The water is cleaned.

Other things are not safe. Motor oils and strong household cleaners are not safe. Pesticides are not safe. They cause water pollution.

Clean up after your pets. Animal droppings have a bad odor. They have germs in them. Insects will come to them. People might step on animal droppings. They get on their shoes and then get inside their home. Suppose you walk your dog. Carry a pooper scooper and bag with you. Clean up after your dog. Suppose you have a cat. Change the kitty litter often.

DO NOT POLLUTE
CAN
THE
LITTER!

Anti-Litter Poster

Life Skill

• I will keep the air, land, and water clean and safe.

Materials: Large paper, markers

Directions: You can help keep your environment clean. Follow the directions below to make a poster that tells people not to litter.

Activity

1. **Write a saying on your paper that tells people not to litter.** Your saying should be something people will remember. Your saying might rhyme.

2. **Decorate your poster.** You might draw a place that does not have litter. You might draw kinds of litter. You might draw a trash can.

3. **Hang your poster in your classroom.**

Lesson 32

Review

Vocabulary

Write a separate sentence using each vocabulary word listed on page 232.

Health Content

1. How is your community kept clean? **page 233**

2. What are kinds of litter? **page 234**

3. What are kinds of water pollution? **page 235**

4. What are kinds of air pollution? **page 235**

5. How can you keep your community clean? **page 236**

Keep the Noise Down

Vocabulary

noise: sounds that make you feel uncomfortable or annoyed.

hearing aid: a small device that makes sounds louder.

decibel: a measure of the loudness of sounds.

ear plugs: plugs put in the ears to block sounds.

ear protectors: coverings worn over the ears to block sounds.

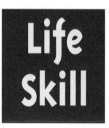

Life Skill

• I will keep noise at a safe level.

Noise is sounds that make you feel uncomfortable or annoyed. The noise from a lawn mower might hurt your ears. The noise from a stereo might make it hard for you to study. You can protect yourself from noise. You can avoid making noise.

The Lesson Objectives

• Explain ways noise harms health.

• Explain how noise makes it hard to study.

• Explain how noise can result in accidents.

• Tell ways to protect your hearing.

Why Do I Need to Keep Noise at a Safe Level?

Noise can harm your health. Suppose you hear loud noise. It can give you a headache. It can make your ears ring and hurt. Loud noises can cause stress. Your heart rate goes up. Your blood pressure goes up. You feel stressed out. It can make you very tired.

Noise can cause hearing loss. *Hearing loss* is being unable to hear some sounds. Some people have hearing loss. They might have been around very loud noise just once. They might have been around loud noise often. The loud noise caused the hearing loss. These people might wear a hearing aid. A **hearing aid** is a small device that makes sounds louder.

Noise can make it hard to study and learn. You study and learn more if it is quiet. Noise makes it hard to think about what you are doing. It makes it hard for you to hear your teacher. You might not get the directions straight. Then you do not do your work the right way. You make mistakes.

Noise stops you from hearing warning sounds to keep you safe. Suppose you listen to headphones while you cross the street. You might not hear a car honk its horn. You might get hit by the car.

Keep the Noise Down

Do you play your music loudly? Do you scream and yell while you play in your yard? You might be bothering other people. Remember, other people hear the noise you make. Do not make loud noise that bothers other people. Do not play loud music when people are sleeping.

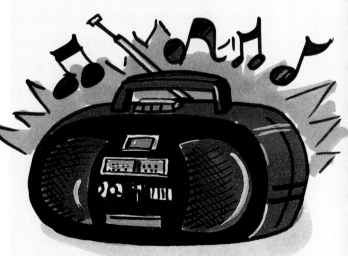

How Can I Protect My Hearing?

A **decibel** (DE·suh·buhl) is a measure of the loudness of sounds. Some sounds are safe. The loudness of talk is 60 decibels. The loudness of a vacuum cleaner is 70 decibels. The loudness of a lawnmower is 85 to 90 decibels. The loudness of rock music at a concert is 115 decibels.

Suppose you are three feet away from someone. The person shouts to you. The loudness of shouting is about 85 decibels. Protect your hearing if loudness is 85 decibels. You can have hearing loss from sounds that loud.

Stay away from loud noises. Keep the sound from TV and music down. Stay away from places with loud noise.

Wear ear plugs or special ear muffs. **Ear plugs** are plugs put in the ears to block sounds. They are made of foam or plastic. Ear protectors block more sound than ear plugs. **Ear protectors** are coverings worn over the ears to block sounds. They look like headphones.

Cover your ears with your hands. Suppose there is a sudden loud noise. You do not have ear plugs or special ear protectors. Put your hands over your ears. Get away from the loud noise.

Cotton Blocks Noise—No Way!

Suppose there is loud noise. Someone says you can put cotton balls in your ears. The person says this will protect hearing. No way! Cotton balls do not block sounds over 85 decibels.

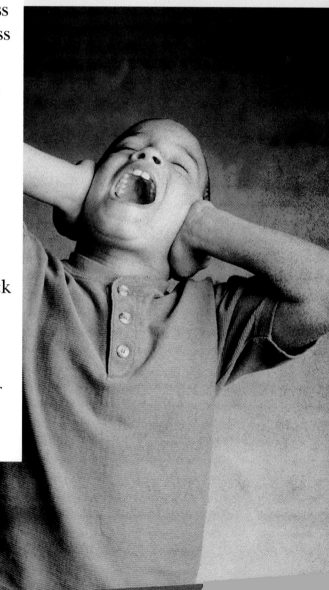

Use... Guidelines for Making Responsible Decisions™

Situation:

You are doing your homework. You also are listening to your favorite radio music program. It is very loud.

Response:

Answer "yes" or "no" to each of the following questions. Explain each answer.

1. Is it healthful to listen to loud music while you do your homework?

2. Is it safe to listen to loud music while you do your homework?

3. Do you follow rules and laws if you listen to loud music while you do your homework?

4. Do you show respect for yourself and others if you listen to loud music while you do your homework?

5. Do you follow your family's guidelines if you listen to loud music while you do your homework?

6. Do you show good character if you listen to loud music while you do your homework?

What is the responsible decision to make?

Lesson 33

Review

Vocabulary

Write a separate sentence using each vocabulary word listed on page 238.

Health Content

1. How can noise harm health? **page 239**

2. How does noise make it hard to study and learn? **page 239**

3. How can noise cause you to get hurt in an accident? **page 239**

4. How can you protect your hearing? **page 240**

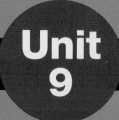
It's a Waste

Vocabulary

resources: things that occur in nature and are used to make other things.

energy: the ability to do work.

landfill: a place where waste is dumped and buried.

precycle: to keep from making trash.

recycle: to change trash so it can be used again.

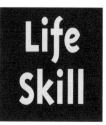

Life Skill

- **I will not waste energy and resources.**

Resources (REE·sohr·sez) are things that occur in nature and are used to make other things. Coal is a resource. It is burned to make electricity. Natural gas is a resource. It is burned to make heat. Electricity and gas are used for energy. **Energy** is the ability to do work.

The Lesson Objectives

- Explain how you can make less trash.
- Discuss how you can save gas and electricity.

How Can I Make Less Trash?

Trash is something that is thrown away. Trash is put into a landfill. A **landfill** is a place where waste is dumped and buried.

There are reasons to make less trash. Resources were used to make products that are trash. These resources could be used in other ways. For example, the more trash there is, the more land that is needed for landfills. Land could be used for something else.

How to precycle To **precycle** is to keep from making trash. Suppose you pack your lunch for school each day. You might put your food in a plastic container. You might put your drink in a thermos. You place these in a lunch box. Each day you bring them home. You wash them and use them again. You do not make trash. Suppose you put your food in aluminum foil. Suppose your drink was in a bottle. Then you put them in a paper sack. You would make trash.

How to recycle To **recycle** is to change trash so it can be used again. Glass bottles, glass jars, and soda pop cans can be used again. There is a place in your community to take them. Do not throw them in the trash.

Keep Up the Green!

It's everyone's job
  to help how they can
To keep our
  environment clean.
To reduce and reuse
  and recycle is the plan
To be healthful and
  keep up the green.

Where do things go when
  you throw them away?
You might think they
  just disappear.
But all of the things
  that you use every day
Have to go somewhere
  from here.

You might think
  there's not very
  much you can do
To keep our
  environment clean.
But everyone can do
  their part—even you,
To recycle and keep
  up the green!

How Can I Save Gas and Electricity?

Energy is the ability to do work. Suppose you use an appliance like a toaster. It takes energy for the toaster to work. Suppose you turn on the lights in your bedroom. It takes energy for them to work.

Suppose you are cold and turn up the heat in your home. The higher the heat is turned the more energy used. Suppose you turn an air conditioner on. It uses more energy than if you used a fan.

There are different kinds of energy. Electricity is used for heat. It is used to make appliances and lights work. Natural gas is used for heat.

Ways to Save Gas and Electricity

- Turn off the lights when you leave a room.

- Turn off the stereo and radio when you are not listening to them.

- Turn off the TV if you are not watching it.

- Turn off your computer and monitor if you are not using them.

- Wear a sweater and use an extra blanket so you can keep heat turned lower.

- Use fans instead of turning the air conditioner to very cold.

Use Your Own Energy

When you want to visit a friend who lives nearby, what do you do? Perhaps you ask a parent or guardian to drive you. But could you walk or ride your bike? If the friend lives near enough that you could get there easily, ask your parents or guardian for permission. You will save energy by saving the gasoline in the car. And you will help your health by getting physical activity.

Lights Out

Life Skill

• I will not waste energy and resources.

Materials: Poster board, markers, scissors

Directions: Make a "Lights Out" hangtag to remind your family to save energy.

CLICK

1. **Cut out a hangtag from poster board.** A hangtag is hung on a doorknob or other knob.

2. **Draw a light bulb and write "Lights Out" on your hangtag.**

3. **Ask your parents or guardian to let you put it on the doorknob.** Family members will see it when they leave the home. It will remind them to turn the lights out.

Activity

Lesson 34

Review

Vocabulary

Write a separate sentence using each vocabulary word listed on page 242.

Health Content

1. How can you make less trash when you take your lunch to school? **page 243**
2. How can you precycle? **page 243**
3. What products can you recycle? **page 243**
4. How can you use your own energy? **page 244**
5. How can you help save gas and electricity? **page 244**

A Friendly Place

Vocabulary

friendly environment: an environment in which people get along, cooperate, and share space.

cooperate: to work well with others toward a goal.

neighborhood: the small area in which you live.

visual environment: everything you see often.

graffiti: writing on property.

Life Skill

● I will help keep my environment friendly.

A **friendly environment** is an environment in which people get along, cooperate, and share space. To **cooperate** (koh·AH·puh·rayt) is to work well with others toward a goal. A friendly environment is healthful. You feel safe and happy when you have a friendly environment. You know that other people respect you.

The Lesson Objectives

● Explain how you can keep your neighborhood looking nice.

● Discuss ways you can enjoy the environment with others.

How Can I Keep My Neighborhood Looking Nice?

Your **neighborhood** is the small area in which you live. Suppose you look around your neighborhood. The **visual environment** is everything you see often. What do you see in your neighborhood? Do you keep your neighborhood looking nice?

Keep your property clean and safe. Suppose you live in an apartment building. Keep the hallway clean. Put your trash in containers. Place your bike where you are asked to put it. Do your part to keep snow shoveled or grass cut.

Suppose you live in a house. Keep the steps to your house clear. Remember, people can trip on toys. Put your bike and other belongings away. Help shovel snow or mow grass.

Improve what is in your neighborhood. Plant flowers, trees, or shrubs. Weed the garden. Put out a bird feeder. Fix things that are broken.

Do not write graffiti. Graffiti (grah·FEE·tee) is writing on property. Do not carve your initials or words on a bench or tree. Do not write or draw in wet concrete.

Clean up after your pets. Use a pooper scooper. Pick up animal droppings and put them in a trash bag.

Show Respect for Neighbors

- Say hello to neighbors you know.
- Do not damage property.
- Do not make loud noises.
- Do not mow grass or play loud music when people are sleeping.

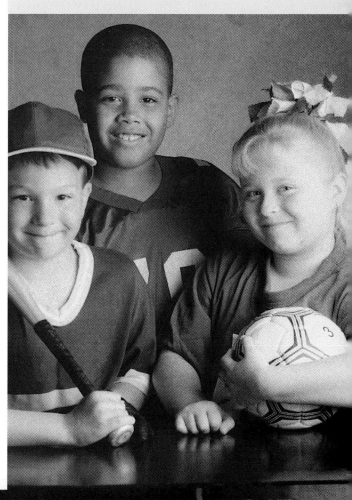

How Can I Enjoy the Environment with Others?

There are many places and activities you can enjoy in your environment. You can plan to spend time with family members and friends. You can enjoy these places and activities with them. You will have less stress when you spend time outdoors in the environment.

Plan a family trip to the zoo. You can learn about many animals and how they live. You can see animals you would not see anywhere else.

You might enjoy visiting a public garden. You can see all kinds of plants. Herbs, roses, and rock gardens are some of the special kinds of gardens you might see.

Plan a picnic at a local park. You might play frisbee or other games in grassy areas. You might walk on a nature trail. You might see trees, animals, birds, and more. If you live near mountains, there might be special views or activities you can enjoy.

You might live near the ocean. You can enjoy the sound of the ocean. You can look for seashells. You might make a seashell collection. Or you might be able to visit an aquarium. An *aquarium* (uh·KWEHR·ee·uhm) is an indoor tank where fish and other water animals live. You can see many kinds of fish, turtles, and eels up close.

Take a Walk in Your Neighborhood

You can take a walk in your neighborhood with members of your family. Get physical activity. Look around at other houses. Notice your neighbors' flowers or other decorations. Wave to or speak with your neighbors. You might notice things you never saw before.

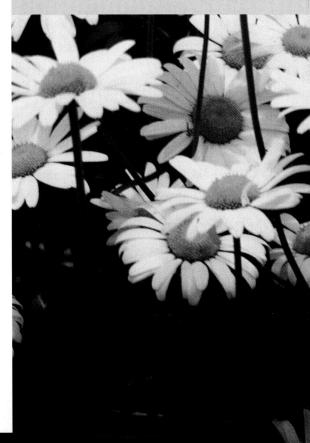

Mural of Places to Enjoy

Activity

Life Skill

- I will help keep my environment friendly.

Materials: Roll of paper, paints, and paint brush

Directions: A mural is a picture that is painted over space. Make a mural with your classmates.

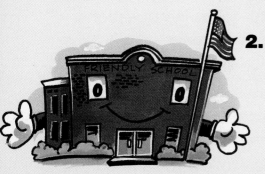

1. **Your teacher will place a long roll of paper on the floor or wall.**

2. **Paint places in the environment to enjoy. Begin at one end of the mural.** Choose what you will paint first. You might paint a flower garden. Then choose something else. You might paint animals in the zoo. You might paint a park or ocean.

Lesson 35

Review

Vocabulary

Write a separate sentence using each vocabulary word listed on page 246.

Health Content

1. How can you keep your property clean and safe? **page 247**

2. What are ways to improve your neighborhood? **page 247**

3. Where are places people write graffitti? **page 247**

4. How can you clean up after pets? **page 247**

5. Where are places to go to enjoy the environment? **page 248**

Unit 9 Review

Health Content

1. What do volunteers in an Adopt-a-Highway Program do? **Lesson 32 page 233**

2. What are ways litter can harm your health? **Lesson 32 page 234**

3. What are ways you can keep your community clean? **Lesson 32 page 236**

4. What are ways noise can make it hard to study? **Lesson 33 page 239**

5. When should you wear hearing protection? **Lesson 33 page 240**

6. What are ways you can precycle? **Lesson 34 page 243**

7. What are products you can recycle? **Lesson 34 page 243**

8. What are ways you can save gas and electricity? **Lesson 34 page 244**

9. What are ways you can keep your neighborhood looking nice? **Lesson 35 page 247**

10. What are ways you can enjoy the environment with others? **Lesson 35 page 248**

Guidelines for Making Responsible Decisions™

There was a big snowstorm last night. Your brother says there is no reason to shovel the snow off the sidewalk. He says it will just snow again. Answer "yes" or "no" to each of the following questions. Explain each answer.

1. Is it healthful to leave the snow on the sidewalk?

2. Is it safe to leave the snow on the sidewalk?

3. Do you follow rules and laws if you leave the snow on the sidewalk?

4. Do you show respect for yourself and others if you leave the snow on the sidewalk?

5. Do you follow your family's guidelines if you leave the snow on the sidewalk?

6. Do you show good character if you leave the snow on the sidewalk?

What is the responsible decision to make?

Vocabulary

Number a sheet of paper from 1–10. Read each definition. Next to each number on your sheet of paper, write the vocabulary word that matches the definition.

litter	energy
water pollution	cooperate
friendly environment	decibel
ear plugs	landfill
resources	ear protectors

1. A place where waste is dumped and buried. **Lesson 32**
2. The ability to do work. **Lesson 34**
3. Plugs put in the ears to block sounds. **Lesson 33**
4. Substances in water that make it unclean and harmful. **Lesson 32**
5. Coverings worn over the ears to block sounds. **Lesson 33**
6. Things that occur in nature and are used to make other things. **Lesson 34**
7. Trash that is thrown on land or in water. **Lesson 32**
8. To work well with others toward a goal. **Lesson 35**
9. A measure of the loudness of sounds. **Lesson 33**
10. An environment in which people get along, cooperate, and share space. **Lesson 35**

Health Literacy

Effective Communication

Make a poster that shows ways to protect yourself from noise. Hang the poster in a noisy place.

Self-Directed Learning

Read a book about how water is made safe to drink. Write a paragraph that explains what you learned.

Critical Thinking

Why is it important for everyone to help keep a community clean?

Responsible Citizenship

Write a one-minute speech that explains how your classmates can precycle. Give the speech for your class.

Multicultural Health

Read a book about outdoor places people enjoy in other countries. Draw a picture of one of these places.

Unit 10

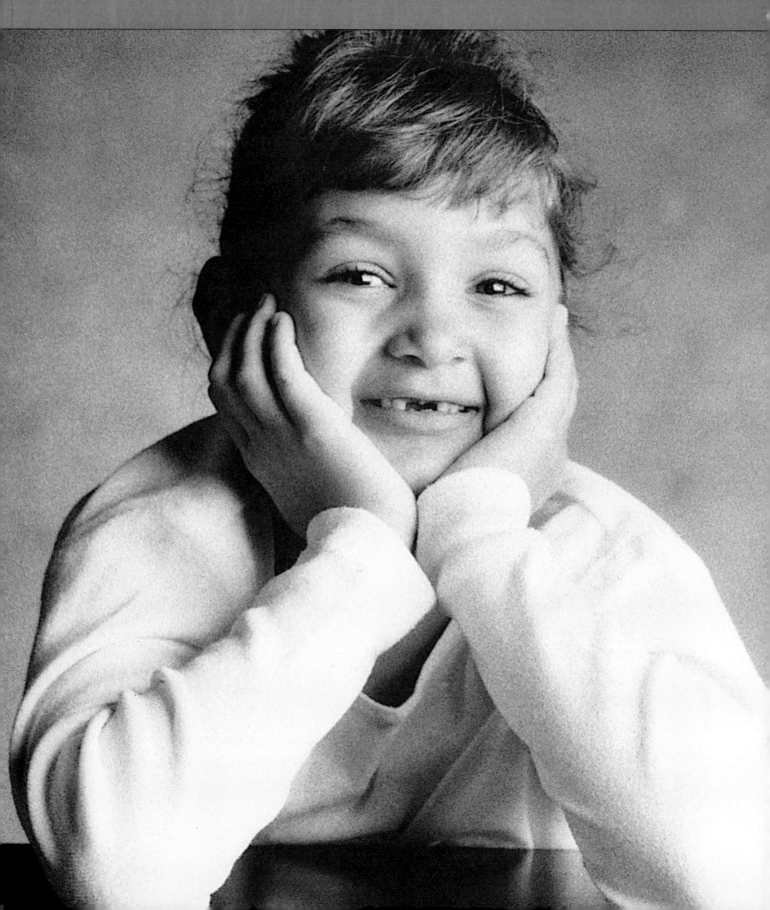

Injury Prevention and Safety

Safe at School, Home, and Play

Vocabulary

rule: a guide to help you do the right thing.

accident: something that is not supposed to happen.

injury: damage or harm done to a person.

poison: a material that can harm you.

fire escape plan: a plan to get out safely if a fire breaks out.

Life Skills

- I will follow safety rules for my home and school.
- I will follow safety rules for weather conditions.

A **rule** is a guide to help you do the right thing. Some rules help keep you safe. They keep you from having an accident. An **accident** (AK·suh·duhnt) is something that is not supposed to happen. You can get injured from an accident. An **injury** is damage or harm done to a person. You can learn safety rules to keep accidents from happening.

The Lesson Objectives

- Tell safety rules when you are at home.
- Tell safety rules when you are at school.
- Tell fire safety rules.
- Tell safety rules when you are outdoors.
- Tell safety rules during bad weather.

What Are Safety Rules to Follow?

Follow safety rules to keep you and others from getting poisoned.

Poison is a material that can harm you. People can breathe in poison. They can swallow poison. They can have poison touch parts of their bodies.

1. Keep the labels on all containers. Do not mark over them. Do not peel them off. Then you will know what is inside each container.

2. Use materials with strong odors only when your parents or guardian are there. Get fresh air when you use these materials.

3. Keep materials in their own containers.

4. Keep all poisons and medicines away from small children.

Follow safety rules to keep you and others from falling.

1. Keep your toys and books put away. You and others can trip over them.

2. Use a stepstool or ladder to reach objects high up. Do not use a chair.

3. Do not run in the house. Walk and watch where you are going.

4. Do not walk on wet floors or floors that have just been waxed.

5. Place rubber mats or rubber stickers in the bathtub.

Follow safety rules to keep you and others safe in school.

1. Keep items off the floor in your classroom.

2. Never run in the hallways or anywhere else unless your teacher says it is okay.

3. Do not walk on wet floors.

4. Do not splash water in the restrooms. The floor might get wet.

5. Wipe up a spill you make.

6. Do not trip someone for fun. It is not fun to break a bone or hit your head!

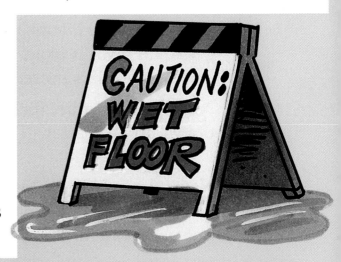

What Are Safety Rules at Home?

Follow safety rules when you take care of your dog.

1. Tell your parents or guardian if your dog is sick or hurt. Do not touch your dog. Your dog might think you are causing the hurt.

2. Play safely with your dog. Do not pull its toys out of its mouth. Do not pull on its ears or tail. Do not play roughly with it. Your dog might bite you by accident.

3. Do not bother your dog while it is eating or sleeping.

Follow safety rules when you are in the kitchen.

1. Follow the rules of your parent or guardian for using the microwave.

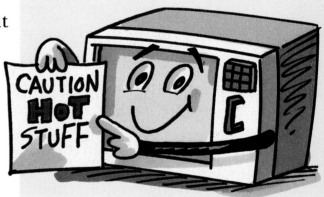

2. Use pot holders when you take items out of the microwave. If an item is very hot, ask an adult to take it out for you.

3. Use a toaster oven, stove, or other appliance only if your parents or guardian say it is okay. Use it only when an adult is there.

4. Never stick a knife, fork, or any object into a toaster. Tell an adult if food gets stuck.

5. Never use a knife unless your parent or guardian says it is okay. Use it only when an adult is watching.

Follow safety rules for using appliances.

You can be injured or start a fire when using appliances.

1. Use an appliance only if your parent or guardian says it is okay. Use it only when an adult is there.

2. Do not use an appliance near water or when you are wet.

What Are Fire Safety Rules?

Follow fire safety rules to prevent a fire.

1. Never play with matches or a lighter.

2. Light candles only if your parents or guardians are there.

3. Use appliances only if your parents or guardian says it is okay. Use them only when an adult is there.

4. Tell an adult if something catches fire in your home.

5. Know where the fire extinguisher is kept. You might need to remind a childsitter if a small fire breaks out.

Follow fire safety rules for getting out in case of fire.

1. Follow your fire escape plan. A **fire escape plan** is a plan to get out safely if a fire breaks out.

2. Do not look around for belongings.

3. Go out a door as your first way out. Feel the door first if it is closed. Do not open the door if it is hot. Put clothes or a sheet along the bottom of the door. Go to a window and yell for help.

4. Crawl out if you can open the door. Cover your mouth and nose.

5. Meet outside at the place your family picked.

6. Do not go back inside for anything.

Your Fire Escape Plan

Fires can burn very quickly. They can fill your house with smoke fast. You might get mixed up or scared if a fire breaks out. You will be less scared if you know a fire escape plan.

- Have your parents or guardian help you.

- Draw a picture of every room in your house.

- Draw arrows to show two ways out of every room.

- Pick a meeting place outside your home.

- Practice the plan with your family twice a year.

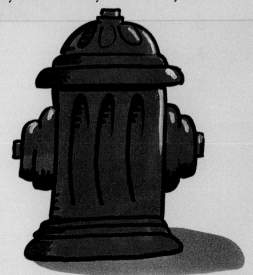

What Are Outdoor Safety Rules?

Follow safety rules when you run outdoors.

1. Be sure your shoelaces are tied.

2. Keep enough space between you and the next person. Sometimes people fall because they trip over each other.

3. Watch where you are going.

4. Do not run around swimming pools or where the pavement is wet and slippery.

5. Do not run in crowded places.

Follow safety rules when you play outdoors.

1. Do not play with equipment that is loose or damaged. Tell an adult.

2. Do not tie ropes to playground equipment. You might get caught in the rope.

3. Do not try stunts or take dares.

4. Do not climb trees.

5. Do not climb power or telephone poles. You might fall or get shocked.

6. Wear safety equipment for sports and other activities. Wear a mouthguard. Wear a helmet when you bike or play football.

Say NO to a Fido You Don't Know!

Never try to make friends with a dog you do not know. Stray dogs might attack and bite you. If a dog starts to chase you, do not run. Stop and stand still. Pretend you are a tree. Put your arms over your face. Try not to look at the dog. The dog should leave in a while.

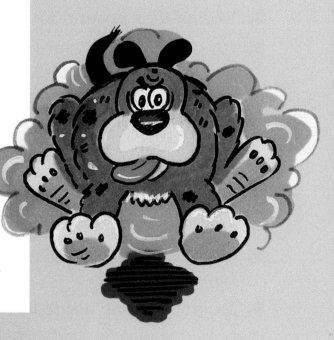

Follow a...
Health Behavior Contract

Copy the health behavior contract on a separate sheet of paper.

DO NOT WRITE IN THIS BOOK.

Name:_____ **Date:** _____

Life Skill: I will follow safety rules for my home and school.

Effect on My Health: Accidents can happen indoors and outdoors. I can have an injury if an accident happens. I can keep many accidents from happening. I can follow safety rules. Then I will not be injured. I will be able to play. I will be able to go to school. I will not cause anyone else to be injured.

My Plan: I will make a calendar. I will list three indoor safety rules. I will list three outdoor safety rules. Each day I will remember safety rules I followed. I will place a check for safety rules I followed for that day.

My Calendar		M	T	W	Th	F	S	S
	Indoor Safety Rules							
	1.							
	2.							
	3.							
	Outdoor Safety Rules							
	1.							
	2.							
	3.							

How My Plan Worked: I will count how many checks I made on my calendar for each safety rule. On the back of my health behavior contract, I will write the safety rule I followed the least. I will write ways I can follow that safety rule.

What Are Safety Rules for Bad Weather?

Follow safety rules if you go out in cold weather.

1. Dress warmly. Dress in layers. Wear mittens instead of gloves. Wear a hat. Cover your mouth with a scarf. The air that reaches your lungs will be warmer.

2. Drink plenty of fluids. Fluids help your body stay at a normal temperature.

3. Keep your skin dry. Change your socks or mittens if they get wet.

4. Go inside and tell an adult if you lose feeling in your nose, fingers, or toes.

Follow safety rules if you go out in hot weather.

1. Wear loose, light-colored clothes.

2. Wear a sunscreen with an SPF (sun protection factor) of 15 or higher.

3. Do not play or run hard. Your body temperature will get hotter.

4. Drink plenty of fluids.

Follow safety rules during a thunderstorm.

Lightning can travel through electrical outlets. Lightning can travel through water and sewer pipes.

1. Do not touch any electrical equipment. Do not use the telephone. Have your parents or guardian unplug televisions and computers.

2. Keep away from sinks, bathtubs, and toilets.

3. Go inside if you are outdoors and you hear thunder or see lightning. Do not wait for rain to start.

Follow safety rules during a flood.

A flood can follow a thunderstorm. A *flood* is the overflow of water onto dry land.

1. Do not wade, play, or swim in flood water. Flood water can contain harmful germs and chemicals. You can get swept away by flood water.

2. Follow your teacher's directions if you are at school. Stay with your teacher or other adult.

Follow safety rules during a tornado.

A tornado can follow a thunderstorm. A *tornado* is a high speed windstorm that is shaped like a funnel.

1. Go to the basement of your home.

2. Stay in the center of the ground floor if your home has no basement.

3. Stay away from windows.

4. Get under heavy furniture.

5. Go indoors if you are outdoors. Lie in a ditch if you cannot get indoors.

6. Follow your teacher's directions if you are at school.

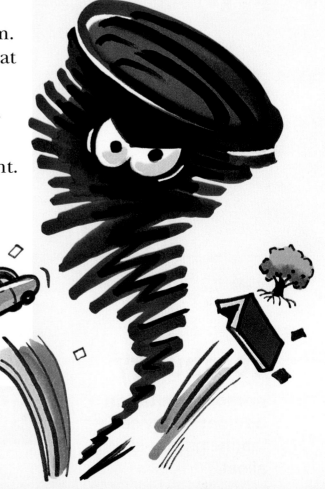

Lesson 36

Review

Vocabulary

Write a separate sentence using each vocabulary word listed on page 254.

Health Content

1. What are safety rules when you are at school? **page 255**

2. What are safety rules when you are at home? **page 256**

3. What are fire safety rules? **page 257**

4. What are safety rules when you are outdoors? **page 258**

5. What are safety rules during bad weather? **pages 260–261**

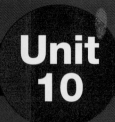
Safe on the Go

Vocabulary

personal flotation device: a device that helps you stay afloat.

safety belt: the lap belt and the shoulder belt.

Life Skills

- I will follow safety rules for biking, walking, and swimming.
- I will follow safety rules for riding in a car.

You can be injured when you ride your bike, take a walk, skate, or swim. You can be injured when you ride in a car or bus. You need to learn safety rules for staying safe when you are on the go.

The Lesson Objectives

- Tell safety rules when you ride a bike.
- Tell safety rules when you walk.
- Tell safety rules when you skate.
- Tell safety rules when you play in the water.
- Tell safety rules when you ride in a car or bus.

How Can I Stay Safe When I Bike?

Follow safety rules when you ride a bike.

1. Always wear a bicycle helmet. A helmet protects you from head injury if you crash or fall. It is the law in some places to wear a helmet. Wear your bicycle helmet correctly. It should not be too tight or too loose.

2. Do not ride in a street or road. Ride on bike paths when possible. Ride on sidewalks only if it is allowed. Ride on the right side. Pass on the left. Slow down when you pass someone. Yell out, "Passing on the left!"

3. Ride your bike only in daylight. Do not ride your bike at dawn, dusk, or night. Bring your bike home when the sun sets.

4. Stop and look both ways if you must cross a street. Wait until no traffic is coming. Walk your bike across the street.

5. Control your bike at all times. Do not ride too fast. Do not ride double. Do not let anyone sit on your handlebars.

6. Wear the right kind of clothing when you ride. Do not wear long dresses, wide-legged pants, or any clothing that could get caught in the bike.

Keep Your Bike in Good Condition

Make sure your brakes work well. Oil moving parts of your bike every few months. Check the tires to see if they have enough air in them. Use a hand pump if you must put air into the tires. Do not put air into bike tires with an air pump at a service station. The pressure inside the air pump is too powerful. The tire could explode and you could get hurt. If you drop the air hose, it could come back up and hit you.

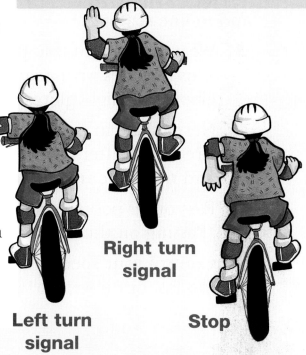

Left turn signal

Right turn signal

Stop

How Can I Stay Safe When I Walk and Skate?

Follow safety rules when you walk.

1. Walk on sidewalks, not in the street. Walk in the street next to the curb if there are no sidewalks. Walk facing the oncoming traffic. Walk single file.

2. Cross streets at corners. Use crosswalks if they are there.

3. Look both ways before crossing a street. Look first to the left, then to the right, and then to the left again. Cross when you are sure no cars are coming.

4. Follow traffic signs and lights.

Follow safety rules when you skate.

This includes rollerskates, skateboards, and in-line skates.

1. Wear equipment that protects you. This includes wrist guards, knee pads, elbow pads, light gloves, and a helmet.

2. Never skate in the street. Cross a street only after you look both ways and no traffic is coming.

3. Pass other people on the left. Yell, "Passing on the left!"

4. Control your speed. Do not skate too fast or on wet surfaces.

Learn How to Fall

Falls will happen when you skate. You can lessen your chance of injury if you learn how to fall.

- Practice falling on soft grass or on a gym mat.

- Crouch down if you are about to fall. You will not fall as far.

- Try to roll instead of sticking out your arms if you fall.

- Try to go limp instead of being stiff.

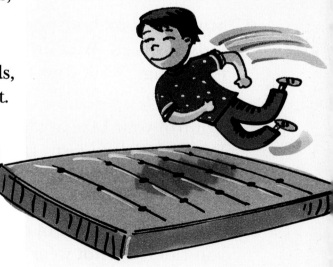

How Can I Stay Safe When I Play in the Water?

Follow safety rules when you swim.

1. Swim with a friend. Do not get in the water by yourself.

2. Swim only when an adult is watching.

3. Do not eat or chew gum while you are swimming. You might choke and breathe in water.

4. Swim in areas marked for swimming. Do not go far out. Do not go past signs that say, "No swimming."

5. Do not swim if you get tired or chilled.

Follow safety rules when you dive.

1. Dive only in places where you are sure it is deep enough. Dive only when an adult is watching.

2. Do not dive near or on top of someone.

Follow safety rules when you ride in a boat.

1. Always wear a personal flotation device. A **personal flotation device** (PUHR·suhn·uhl floh·TAY·shuhn di·VYS) is a device that helps you stay afloat. Wear it even if you know how to swim. A life jacket is best.

2. Do not hang over the boat.

3. Do not push others.

Good "Water Manners"

You know good table manners. You need to know good water manners. It is okay to have fun when you swim, dive, or ride in a boat. But you can hurt someone if you do not use water manners. Do not push, dunk, or shove others. Never push anyone off a diving board. Go down one at a time on a slide. Do not hit anyone with water toys. Do not run around a pool.

Right Way, Wrong Way

Choose a safety rule in this lesson. Draw a picture that shows a person following the rule. Draw a picture that shows a person who is not following the rule. Draw a big red circle around the wrong way. Draw a red slash through the picture.

How Can I Stay Safe When I Ride in a Car?

Follow safety rules when you ride in a car, truck, or van.

1. Wear a safety belt every time you ride in a car, truck, or van. A **safety belt** is the lap belt and the shoulder belt. A safety belt holds you in your seat during a crash. It keeps you from being forced against the inside of the car. It keeps you from being thrown from the car.

2. Wear a safety belt correctly. It should be snug but not tight. The shoulder belt should not go across your neck or under your arm. It should go across your chest.

3. Ride in the back seat. You are safer if the car crashes. You will not hit your head against the dashboard.

4. Put your seat as far back as possible if you must ride in the front seat. Wear your safety belt!

5. Do not ride in the back of a pickup truck. Do not ride on the floor of a station wagon or van.

6. Lock your door when you are inside. The door will not open in an accident.

7. Get in and out on the curb side. You will not get hit by traffic.

Ride with a Responsible Driver

Do not ride with a driver who has been drinking alcohol. Suppose you are at a friend's house or at a party. An adult or teen offers to drive you home. Call your parents or guardian to come and get you if:

- You have seen the person who will drive drinking alcohol.

- You smell alcohol on the breath of the person who will drive.

How Can I Stay Safe When I Ride the School Bus?

Follow safety rules when you get on or off the school bus.

1. Stand at least three giant steps away from the street curb when you are waiting for the school bus.

2. Wait for the driver to signal you if you cross the street to get on the school bus.

3. Look both ways before you step off the school bus if you must cross the street.

Follow safety rules when you ride a school bus.

1. Stay in your seat.

2. Stay quiet. Yelling, screaming, and throwing things will bother the driver.

3. Keep the aisle safe. Do not put anything in the aisle. Do not trip people.

Lesson 37

Review

Vocabulary

Write a separate sentence using each vocabulary word listed on page 262.

Health Content

1. What are safety rules when you ride a bike? **page 263**

2. What are safety rules when you walk? **page 264**

3. What are safety rules when you skate? **page 264**

4. What are safety rules when you play in the water? **page 265**

5. What are rules when you ride in a car or school bus? **pages 266–267**

Safe Around People

Vocabulary

loving actions: actions that show your special feelings for someone.

unloving actions: actions that harm other people.

violence: harm done to yourself, others, or property.

stranger: someone you do not know well.

unsafe touch: a touch that is not right.

Life Skills

- I will protect myself from people who might harm me.
- I will follow safety rules to protect myself from violence.

Most of the people around you are loving and kind. But some of the people around you are not kind. They might harm you. You need to know how you can stay safe around people who might want to harm you.

The Lesson Objectives

- Tell safety rules when you are home with someone besides your parents or guardian.
- Tell safety rules when you are walking or playing away from home.
- Tell safety rules to stay safe from strangers in cars.
- Tell what to do if someone gives you an unsafe touch.

How Can I Protect Myself from People Who Might Harm Me?

Loving feelings are feelings you have toward someone you care about. Love can be more than a feeling. Love is also a way of acting. **Loving actions** are actions that show your special feelings for someone. When you love someone, you show it. You might hug your parents or guardian. You might help your best friend with homework. You might play with your pet.

People do not always have loving actions. They sometimes have unloving actions. **Unloving actions** are actions that harm other people. Unloving actions are not kind. They are cruel or angry or mean. Unloving actions might be violence. **Violence** is harm done to yourself, others, or property.

There are many adults around you most of the time. You know some of these people well. Some of the people around you might be friends of your parents. Other adults around you are strangers. A **stranger** (STRAYN·juhr) is someone you do not know well.

Some adults might want to harm you. They might be strangers. But they might be adults you know. You can protect yourself from people who might harm you. You can follow safety rules to protect yourself from violence.

Who Can You Trust If You Are Lost?

An adult who works in a store Make sure the adult is wearing a badge with his or her name and the name of the store.

A lifeguard if you are lost at the beach

An adult at the "Lost and Found" if you are at an amusement park Make sure the adult is wearing a badge with his or her name and the name of the park.

A police officer Make sure the police officer is wearing a badge and a uniform.

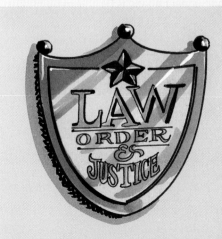

How Can I Stay Safe at Home?

Suppose you are at home with an older brother or sister or a childsitter. You can be safe when you are home without your parents or guardian.

Follow safety rules when you answer the phone.

1. Say "hello" when you answer. Never say your name or your family name. The caller might ask, "Who is this?" You should answer, "Who are you calling?"

2. Never give your address or telephone number. The caller might ask, "What number is this?" You should answer, "What number did you call?"

3. Never tell anyone your parents or guardians are not home. Say, "They cannot come to the phone right now." Ask if you can take a message.

4. Never answer other questions a caller might ask.

5. Never agree to buy anything over the telephone.

6. HANG UP if the caller bothers you or says something mean or dirty.

Follow safety rules if someone comes to the door.

1. Keep the doors locked at all times.

2. Stay inside your house.

3. Do not let anyone into your home. It does not matter if:

   - you know the person.
   - the person is wearing a uniform.
   - the person says your parents or guardian said it was okay.

Let a person into your home only if your parents or guardian tell you it is okay.

4. Call your parents or guardian if a stranger shows up at your home. Call 9-1-1 or the police if you cannot get your parents or guardian.

How Can I Stay Safe While Walking or Playing?

There might be a stranger near where you are walking or playing. It might be the first time you have seen this stranger. Or you might have seen this stranger many times. No matter how many times you have seen the person, this person is a stranger. Protect yourself from violence.

Follow safety rules while walking or playing.

1. Walk and play with friends. You are safer when you are with other children.

2. Know a place nearby where you can run and find an adult you trust.

3. Do not play alone in an empty field or an empty house.

4. Do not go close to a stranger to take candy, money, or toys. Stay far enough away so that a stranger cannot touch you.

5. Do not go anywhere with a stranger. Even if a stranger offers to take you to your parents, do not go.

6. Run away as fast as you can if a stranger bothers you. Run to your home or school or to a store. Yell as you run. You will get the attention of other people.

7. Tell your parents or guardian about any stranger who bothers you.

Get a Good Look

You might be scared if a stranger bothers you. But try to notice how the stranger looks. Your parents, guardian, or teacher might call the police if you are bothered by a stranger. Your description might help the police find the stranger. The police might ask you these questions:

- What color hair did the stranger have?
- How old was the stranger?
- What was the stranger wearing?
- Was the stranger in a car?
- What color was the car?
- Can you remember the license plate number?

How Can I Be Safe from Strangers in Cars?

There might be a stranger in a car driving down the street where you walk. The stranger might follow you. The stranger might stop his or her car and try to talk to you. You can never tell if a stranger in a car is kind or cruel. Protect yourself from violence.

Follow safety rules around strangers in a car.

1. Do not go close to a car in which there is a stranger.

2. Do not accept candy, toys, or money from a stranger. A stranger might try to get you close to the car by offering you such things.

3. Do not walk over to a car to answer a question or to give directions.

4. Do not let a stranger in a car follow you. Turn and run in the opposite direction.

5. Make a noise if a stranger in a car follows you. Other people will hear you and come to see what is wrong.

6. Run to a safe place. Run home if it is near or into a store. Some homes have a sign in a window. The sign might read, "Safe Home." An adult lives there who will help you. Go to such a house if someone follows you.

Pass on This Ride

Is there ever a time when you should get into a car with a stranger? Suppose a stranger tells you that your parent or guardian has been in an accident. The stranger says he or she will take you to the hospital. Suppose a bad storm is coming or it is raining hard. The stranger says he or she will take you home. Should you accept? NO! **NEVER GET INTO A CAR WITH A STRANGER!**

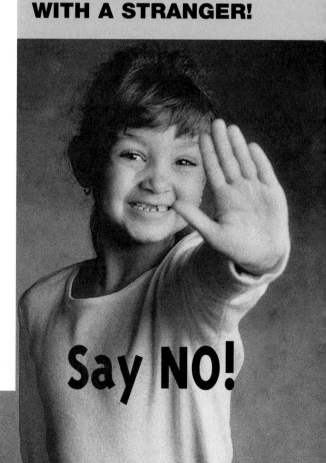

Say NO!

What Is Unsafe Touch?

Suppose you are alone with a friend of your parents or guardian. Your parents or guardian trust this person to look after you. The person touches a private part of your body. The person tells you not to tell your parents or guardian or you will get in trouble.

The person has given you an unsafe touch. An **unsafe touch** is a touch that is not right. This person has shown violence toward you. The person has harmed you.

You have a right not to be harmed. This person has no right to give you an unsafe touch. You will NOT get into trouble if you tell. You are not to blame. You did not do anything wrong.

Follow these rules if a person gives you an unsafe touch.

1. Tell the person to stop touching you.

2. Yell as loud as you can, if the person does not stop touching you.

3. Run away from this person.

4. Tell your parents or guardian. If they are not around, tell another adult you trust.

Lesson 38

Review

Vocabulary

Write a separate sentence using each vocabulary word listed on page 268.

Health Content

1. Who can you trust if you are lost? **page 269**

2. What are safety rules when you answer the phone? When a person knocks at the door? **page 270**

3. What are safety rules when you are walking or playing? **page 271**

4. What are safety rules to stay safe from strangers in cars? **page 272**

5. What should you do if someone gives you an unsafe touch? **page 273**

SAFE from Weapons

Vocabulary

weapon: an object used to harm someone.

gang: a group of people who do violent things.

graffiti: writing on property.

Life Skills

- I will stay away from gangs.
- I will **not carry a weapon.**

You might hang out with a group of friends. You choose friends who make responsible decisions. You and your friends do not hurt others. You and your friends do not carry weapons. A **weapon** is an object used to harm someone. Some groups of people do hurt others. They do carry weapons. You need to learn how to stay safe from these people. You need to learn how to stay safe from weapons.

The Lesson Objectives

- Tell ways gang members are violent.
- Tell ways you can stay away from gangs.
- Tell why you should not pretend to have a weapon.
- Tell steps to take if you find a weapon.

How Are Gang Members Violent?

There might be gangs in your neighborhood. A **gang** is a group of people who do violent things. A gang has a name. Gang members hang out only with one another. They hang out in certain places. They wear certain colors or clothes to show they are members of the same gang. Gang members write graffiti. **Graffiti** (grah·FEE·TEE) is writing on property. This is their way of communicating with other members and other gangs.

Gang members act in violent ways. They do things that are against the law. They carry weapons. Gang members often carry knives and handguns. They get into fights with members of other gangs. Gang members often sell and use drugs that are against the law. They rob and hurt people who are not gang members.

To join a gang, people have to do what the gang members tell them to do. They might be told to steal, buy drugs, or harm someone. After a person joins a gang, the person might find it hard to drop out of the gang. Other gang members might harm a person who tries to drop out of a gang. They might harm members of the person's family.

Ways to Stay Away from Gangs

1. Stay away from gang members.

2. Stay away from places where gang members hang out.

3. Do not be friends with a person who belongs to a gang.

4. Say NO if you are asked to join a gang.

5. Tell your parents or guardian if someone asks you to join a gang.

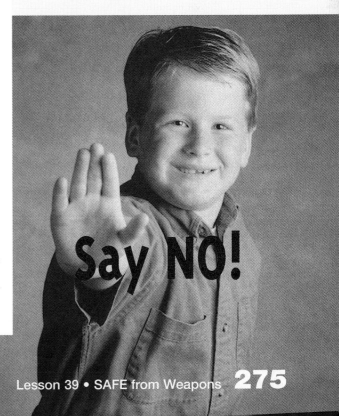

Say NO!

How Can I Be Safe from Weapons?

A weapon is an object used to harm someone. A weapon might be a gun or a knife. It might be a baseball bat. A person might be harmed on purpose by a weapon. Sometimes a person is around someone with a weapon and is harmed by accident. Stay away from weapons. Stay away from people who carry weapons. Never touch a weapon.

Sometimes people pretend they are going to use a knife or a gun. Or they might pretend that a toy gun is a real gun. This is dangerous. Other people might not know they are pretending. Other people with real weapons might harm them.

Follow school rules about weapons. Do not bring weapons to school. Do not bring toy weapons to school. Tell a responsible adult if someone at your school has a weapon. These rules keep people safe in your school.

Follow the SAFE rule if you find a weapon. Follow the SAFE rule if you see a person with a weapon.

S—Stop.

A—Avoid going near the weapon.

F—Find an adult.

E—Explain what you saw.

Real or Make-Believe?

Some guns look like toys. Sometimes it is hard to tell the difference. You might think a gun is a toy when it is real. Never touch a gun even if you think it is a toy. Follow the SAFE rules.

How Can You Protect Yourself and Others?

Suppose you are at a friend's house. Your friend shows you a gun in a drawer. She says it has no bullets in it. She asks you to pull the trigger for fun. Why is this a wrong decision? Why do you need to tell your parent or guardian what happened?

Use... Guidelines for Making Responsible Decisions™

Situation:

A friend is thinking about joining a gang. This friend says joining a gang will bring new friends. This friend starts wearing the colors of the gang. The friend tells you that you should join the gang too.

Response:

Write "yes" or "no" to each of the following questions. Explain each answer.

1. Is it healthful to join a gang?
2. Is it safe to join a gang?
3. Do you follow rules and laws if you join a gang?
4. Do you show respect for yourself and others if you join a gang?
5. Do you follow your family's guidelines if you join a gang?
6. Do you show good character if you join a gang?

What is the responsible decision to make?

Lesson 39

Review

Vocabulary

Write a separate sentence using each vocabulary word listed on page 274.

Health Content

1. What are ways in which gang members are violent? **page 275**
2. What are ways you can stay away from gangs? **page 275**
3. Why should you not pretend to have a weapon? **page 276**
4. What are SAFE steps to follow if you find a weapon? **page 276**
5. What should you do if you think you see a toy gun? **page 276**

Guide to First Aid

Vocabulary

accident:
something that is not
supposed to happen.

first aid: the quick
care given to a
person who has
been injured or
suddenly becomes ill.

emergency: a
situation in which
help is needed quickly.

9-1-1: a phone
number to get help
for an emergency.

first aid kit:
supplies needed
to give first aid.

Life Skill

• I will be skilled in
first aid.

No matter how careful you are, accidents
happen. An **accident** (AK·suh·duhnt) is
something that is not supposed to happen.
A person who is injured might need your help.
You need to know how to get help for an
injured person. You might need to give first aid.
First aid is the quick care given to a person
who has been injured or suddenly becomes ill.

The Lesson Objectives

• Tell rules for helping an injured person.

• Tell rules for calling for help.

• Tell first aid steps for minor injuries.

What Are Rules for Helping an Injured Person?

Suppose you and a friend are riding bikes. Your friend loses control of the bike. Your friend falls. Your friend's leg hurts a lot. It might be broken. What would you do?

Follow rules for helping an injured person.

1. Stay calm. You can think clearly when you are calm.

2. Never move a person who is injured. Moving the person might make the injury worse.

3. Get help fast! Try to get an adult. Send a friend for help or yell for help. If you must leave, tell the injured person where you are going. Tell the person you will be back quickly with help.

4. Cover the person with a blanket or jacket if you have one. The person needs to stay warm.

Always tell your parents, guardian, teacher, or other responsible adult about any injury.

A small injury can turn into a big one. Suppose you hit your head and feel okay. Later you get sick. An adult can tell a doctor that you hit your head. The doctor will know how to treat you.

Emergency!

An **emergency** is a situation in which help is needed quickly. You must tell a responsible adult RIGHT AWAY. Get help quickly if a person:

- has a hard time breathing or stops breathing.
- has bad chest pain.
- has swallowed poison.
- has bleeding that will not stop.
- coughs or vomits blood.
- might have a broken bone.
- has very bad pain.
- passes out.

Be on the safe side: Get help if you are not sure whether it is an emergency. You will not get in trouble. You are doing the right thing.

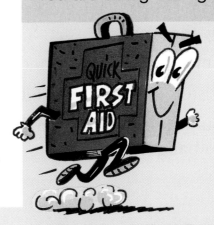

What Are Rules for Calling for Help?

Suppose you are at home with your aunt. Your aunt says she feels dizzy. She passes out. No other adult is in the home. What would you do?

You should tell another adult right away if the adult lives close to you. Call your parents or guardian if they can be reached by phone. Call a neighbor your parents or guardian trust.

Call the special emergency phone number for help. **9-1-1** is a phone number to get help for an emergency. You also can call 0 for an operator.

Follow rules for making an emergency phone call.

1. Call 9-1-1 or 0.

2. Try to speak calmly. You might be upset in an emergency. But try to remember that the injured person needs you to speak calmly to get help.

3. Give your name and address. Your address should be written by the phone.

4. Tell what has happened.

5. Listen to what you are told to do.

6. Stay on the phone until you are told to hang up.

First Aid Kit

Always have a first aid kit in your home. A **first aid kit** is supplies needed to give first aid. You can buy one at a pharmacy or the American Red Cross. Your first aid kit should contain:

- Cold pack
- Gauze pads
- Roller gauze
- Bandage
- Scissors
- Adhesive tape
- Triangular bandage
- Disposable gloves
- Rescue blanket
- Thermometer
- Face mask with one-way valve
- Flashlight
- Extra batteries
- Hot water bottle
- Soap
- Sunscreen
- Syrup of ipecac
- Cotton swabs
- Cotton balls

What Is First Aid for Bleeding?

First Aid for a Small Cut or a Scrape

A *cut* is a break in the skin. A *scrape* is the tearing or wearing away of skin. An adult usually can treat a small cut or scrape. Your parent or guardian might show you how to treat them. No matter how small the cut or scrape, always tell your parent, guardian, or other adult.

1. Clean the cut with soap and water. This removes dirt and germs.

2. Press gently on the cut with a clean cloth or tissue. This helps stop the bleeding.

3. Cover the cut with an adhesive bandage when the bleeding stops. If the cut is too big for an adhesive bandage, the person might need to see a doctor.

4. Wear throw-away gloves if you are helping someone else who has a cut.

First Aid for a Nosebleed

Nosebleeds can have many causes. Tell an adult right away if you get a nosebleed.

1. Sit down and lean forward.

2. Pinch your nostrils shut for ten minutes. Do not blow your nose.

3. Breathe through your mouth. Spit out any blood.

Keep Out the Germs

Some people have germs in their blood. They might not know they have germs. Wear throw-away gloves if you touch someone else's blood. Do not touch your eyes, nose, or mouth while you are helping someone who is bleeding. Do not eat or drink while you are helping someone who is bleeding. Wash your hands with soap and water when you take off the gloves.

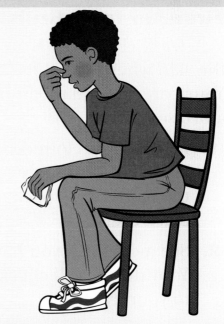

Sit down and lean forward for a nosebleed.

What Is First Aid for Burns and Bruises?

First Aid for a Minor Burn

Suppose you take a dish out of the microwave oven. The dish is very hot. You burn your hand. A *burn* is harm to the body caused by heat. Always tell an adult if you get burned. An adult can treat a burn if it is minor. A minor burn is not serious. Your parent or guardian might show you how to treat a minor burn.

1. Place the burned area under cold water or run cold water over the burn. You also can put ice in a plastic bag and hold it over the area.

2. Pat the area dry.

3. Cover the area with a clean bandage.

First Aid for a Bruise

A *bruise* (BROOZ) is an area under the skin where blood has collected. Your parent or guardian might treat a bruise or black eye.

1. Place a cold cloth or ice pack on the bruise for ten minutes. Do not put the cloth or ice pack directly on a black eye.

2. See a doctor if you have a black eye. Your doctor will check for damage to your eye.

GET HELP!

Tell an adult RIGHT AWAY if someone's clothes catch on fire or someone is splashed with very hot liquid. Call 9-1-1 or 0 if you cannot find an adult.

When Is a Burn Serious?

A serious burn can be caused by very hot liquids or a bad sunburn. A doctor needs to treat a burn that swells, blisters, or is very painful. An adult should decide whether a burn is serious.

GET HELP!

If you think someone has broken a bone, keep the person still. Do not move the person. Do not touch the part that might be broken. Tell an adult RIGHT AWAY. Call 9-1-1 or 0 if you cannot find an adult.

What Is First Aid for Stings and Bites?

First Aid for an Insect Sting

Some people are allergic to certain kinds of insect stings. Allergic means the person has a harmful reaction. A person who is allergic might have trouble breathing. The part of the body that was stung might swell. The person might need emergency help. Always tell an adult if you are stung.

1. Ask an adult for help.

2. Use a fingernail to flick out a bee's stinger. Do not use tweezers.

3. Run cold water or put ice over the area.

4. Tell an adult RIGHT AWAY if later you feel dizzy or short of breath.

First Aid for an Animal Bite

Animal bites can break the skin. They can cause bruising. They can make deep holes in the skin. You can get germs from animal bites. Always tell an adult if you get an animal bite. Tell an adult even if it is your pet. Tell an adult even if the bite seems small.

1. Treat the bite like a cut or scrape if it is minor.

2. Your parents or guardian will take you to a doctor if there is a deep hole in your skin. You can get a serious infection from germs deep in your skin.

Rashes from Plants

Some people are allergic to plants such as poison ivy. The person's skin might itch, burn, and turn red. Stay away from plants to which you are allergic. If you touch them, wash your skin with soap and water right away. Do not use soap that has oil or greasy materials. Put rubbing alcohol on your skin and rinse. If you get a rash, do not scratch. Use an over-the-counter product to ease the itching.

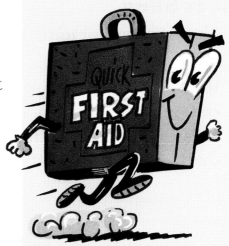

My Quick First Aid Guide

Small Cut or Scrape

1. Clean the cut with soap and water.

2. Press gently on the cut with a clean cloth or tissue.

3. Cover the cut with an adhesive bandage when the bleeding stops.

4. Wear throw-away gloves if you are helping someone else who has a cut.

Minor Burn

1. Place the burned area under cold water or run cold water over the burn.

2. Pat the area dry.

3. Cover the area with a clean bandage.

Insect Sting

1. Use a fingernail to flick out a bee's stinger.

2. Run cold water or put ice over the area. Tell an adult RIGHT AWAY if you feel dizzy or short of breath.

Bruise or Black Eye

1. Place a cold cloth or ice pack on the bruise for ten minutes. Do not put the cloth or ice pack directly on a black eye.

2. See a doctor if you have a black eye.

Nosebleed

1. Sit down and lean forward.

2. Pinch your nostrils shut for ten minutes. Do not blow your nose.

3. Breathe through your mouth. Spit out any blood.

4. Wear throw-away gloves if you are helping someone else who has a nosebleed.

Animal Bite

1. Treat like a cut or scrape if it is minor.

2. Your parents or guardian will take you to a doctor if there is a deep hole in your skin.

First Aid Flash Cards

Life Skill

• I will be skilled in first aid.

Materials: Index cards, pencil

Directions: Do this activity with a partner to help you learn first aid skills.

Activity

1. **Copy each box on page 284 onto an index card.** Copy one box to one card. Do not put the name of the injury.

2. **Copy the name of the injury to the other side of each index card.**

3. **Hold the cards.** Show the side with the name of the injury to your partner. Your partner will say the first aid steps for that injury.

4. **Take turns holding up the cards and saying the first aid steps.**

Lesson 40

Review

Vocabulary

Write a separate sentence using each vocabulary word listed on page 278.

Health Content

1. What are rules for helping an injured person? **page 279**
2. What should you do if you are not sure whether a situation is an emergency? **page 279**
3. What are rules for calling for help? **page 280**
4. Why should you wear gloves when you touch someone else's blood? **page 281**
5. What is first aid for cuts and scrapes; nosebleeds; minor burns; bruises; insect stings; and animal bites? **page 284**

Unit 10 Review

Health Content

1. What are safety rules to keep you safe from falling? **Lesson 36 page 255**

2. What are safety rules to follow when you are in the kitchen? **Lesson 36 page 256**

3. What are safety rules to follow when you ride a bike? **Lesson 37 page 263**

4. What are safety rules to follow when you swim? **Lesson 37 page 265**

5. Who can you trust if you are lost? **Lesson 38 page 269**

6. What are safety rules to follow while walking or playing? **Lesson 38 page 271**

7. How are gang members violent? **Lesson 39 page 275**

8. What is the SAFE rule to follow if you find a weapon? **Lesson 39 page 276**

9. What are rules to follow when making an emergency phone call? **Lesson 40 page 280**

10. Why is it important to wear gloves if you touch someone else's blood? **Lesson 40 page 281**

Guidelines for Making Responsible Decisions™

Several classmates start to write graffiti on the school wall. They dare you to join in. Answer "yes" or "no" to each of the following questions. Explain each answer.

1. Is it healthful to write graffiti on the school wall?

2. Is it safe to write graffiti on the school wall?

3. Do you follow rules and laws if you write graffiti on the school wall?

4. Do you show respect for yourself and others if you write graffiti on the school wall?

5. Do you follow your family's guidelines if you write graffiti on the school wall?

6. Do you show good character if you write graffiti on the school wall?

What is the responsible decision to make?

Vocabulary

Number a sheet of paper from 1–10. Read each definition. Next to each number on your sheet of paper, write the vocabulary word that matches the definition.

violence	injury
personal flotation device	gang
emergency	9-1-1
safety belt	poison
unsafe touch	weapon

1. The lap belt and the shoulder belt. **Lesson 37**
2. A touch that is not right. **Lesson 38**
3. A material that can harm you. **Lesson 36**
4. Harm done to yourself, others, or property. **Lesson 38**
5. Damage or harm done to a person. **Lesson 36**
6. An object used to harm someone. **Lesson 39**
7. A situation in which help is needed quickly. **Lesson 40**
8. A group of people who do violent things. **Lesson 39**
9. A phone number to get help for an emergency. **Lesson 40**
10. A device that helps you stay afloat. **Lesson 37**

Health Literacy

Effective Communication

Draw a picture showing safety rules to follow when riding a bike. Hang the picture in your classroom.

Self-Directed Learning

Check your local library to get information on gangs. Make a safety list on ways to stay away from gangs. Explain why these are important for your safety.

Critical Thinking

Why do you need to know rules now to follow in case of an emergency? Answer the question on a separate sheet of paper.

Responsible Citizenship

Make a poster that shows safety rules to follow at school. Hang the poster in your classroom.

Multicultural Health

Check at your local library to find out if other countries have a 9-1-1 number to call in case of an emergency.

Glossary

Sound	As in	Symbol	Example
ă	cat, tap	a	allergy (AL·uhr·jee)
ā	may, same	ay	coordination (koh·AWR·duh·NAY·shuhn)
a	wear, dare	ehr	marijuana (MEHR·uh·WAH·nuh)
ä	father, top	ah	orthodontist (or·thuh·DAHN·tist)
ar	car, park	ar	arteries (AR·tuh·reez)
ch	chip, touch	ch	childhood (CHYLD·hood)
ě	bet, test	e	independence (IN·duh·PEN·duhnts)
ē	pea, need	ee	anemia (un·NEE·MEE·uh)
er	perk, hurt	er	pituitary (puh·TOO·uh·TER·ee)
g	go, big	g	disability (DI·suh·BI·luh·tee)
ĭ	tip, live	i	cilia (SI·lee·uh)
ī	side, by	y, eye	carbohydrates (kar·boh·HY·drayts)
j	job, edge	j	agility (uh·JI·luh·tee)
k	cook, ache	k	puncture (PUHNK·cher) wound
ō	bone, know	oh	aerobic (uhr·OH·bik) exercise
ô	more, pour	or	hormones (HOR·mohnz)
ȯ	saw, all	aw	alcoholism (AL·kuh·HAW·LI·zuhm)
oi	coin, toy	oy	steriods (STEHR·oydz)
ou	out, now	ow	power (POW·er)
s	see, less	s	cholesteriol (kuh·LES·tuh·rohl)
sh	she, mission	sh	physician (fuh·ZI·shun)
ŭ	cup, dug	uh	fungi (FUHN·jy)
u	wood, pull	u	bully (BUL·ee)
ü	rule, union	oo	nutrients (NOO·tree·uhntz)
w	we, away	w	water (WAH·ter)
y	you, yard	yu	circulation (sur·kyuh·LAY·shun)
z	zone, raise	z	veins (VAYNZ)
zh	vision, measure	zh	decision (di·SI·zhuhn)
ə	around, mug	uh	vitamins (VY·tuh·muhnz)

A

9-1-1: a phone number to get help for an emergency.

accident (AK·suh·duhnt): something that is not supposed to happen.

addiction (uh·DIK·shuhn): letting a drug or habit control you.

adopt: to bring a child from other parents into your family.

Adopt-a-Highway Program: a program in which volunteers pick up trash to keep highways clean.

advertisement (AD·vuhr·TYZ·muhnt): a paid announcement.

aerobic (uhr·OH·bik) **exercise:** exercise that raises your heart rate and causes you to need a lot of air.

agility (uh·JI·luh·tee): the ability to change directions quickly.

AIDS: an illness in which the body cannot fight diseases.

air pollution: substances in the air that make it unsafe to breathe.

alcohol: a drug found in some beverages that slows down the body.

allergen: a substance that causes the body to overreact.

allergy (A·luhr·jee): the body's overreaction to a substance.

allergy (A·luhr·jee) **medicine:** helps get rid of itchy eyes and runny noses.

allowance (uh·LOW·uhnts): an amount of money your parents or guardian give you to spend.

analgesic (a·nuhl·JEE·zik): helps get rid of pain.

antacid: helps get rid of stomach upset.

antibiotic (an·ti·by·AH·tik) **ointment:** kills germs in cuts and scrapes.

antibody (AN·ti·bah·dee): a substance in your blood that kills germs.

anti-perspirant (an·tee·PUHR·spuh·ruhnt): a product used under the arms to reduce perspiration.

appointment: a time when you can see the doctor.

aquarium (uh·KWEHR·ee·uhm): an indoor tank where fish and other water animals live.

arteries (AHR·tuh·reez): blood vessels that take blood away from your heart.

arthritis (ar·THRY·tuhs): a condition in which joints become swollen and sore.

asthma (AZ·muh): a condition in which the air passages become narrow.

289

B

bacteria (bak·TIR·ee·uh): one-celled germs.

balance: the ability to keep from falling.

beta-endorphins (BAY·tuh·en·DOR·fuhns): substances that make you feel good.

bifocals (BY·FOH·kuhlz): a kind of eyeglasses that allow a person to see nearby objects through one part and faraway objects through another part.

blood vessels: tubes that carry blood.

body defenses: ways your body protects you from germs.

body system: a group of organs that work together to do a certain job.

bowel movement: the movement of solid waste out of your body.

Braille (BRAYL): a way of writing with raised dots that blind people can touch to read.

brain: an organ that receives and sends messages to all your body parts.

brainstorm: to write down all the ideas you think of.

bruise (BROOZ): an area under the skin where blood has collected.

bully: a person who tries to frighten or hurt someone who is younger or smaller.

burn: harm to the body caused by heat.

C

caffeine: a stimulant found in chocolate and some beverages.

call number: a number that tells you where the book is in the library.

cancer: a disease in which harmful cells grow.

carbohydrates (kahr·boh·HY·drayts): nutrients that supply the main source of energy for your body.

carbon dioxide (KAR·buhn dy·AHK·SYD): a gas that is a waste product of your cells.

cavity (KA·vuh·tee): a hole in the enamel of a tooth.

CD-ROM (SEE·DEE·RAHM): a computer disc that stores computer programs.

cell: the smallest living part of a person's body.

checkup: an examination of your body.

chore: a small job.

chronic (KRAH·nik) **disease:** a disease that lasts a long time.

cilia: tiny hairs that line the air passages.

circulatory (SUHR·kyuh·luh·TOR·ee) **system:** made up of organs that move blood throughout your body.

cocaine (koh·KAYN): a stimulant made from the leaves of the coca bush.

commercial (kuh·MUHR·shuhl): an ad on radio or television.

communicable (kuh·MYOO·ni·kuh·buhl) **disease:** a disease that can be spread to people from people, animals, and the environment.

community: the place where the people around you live.

conditioner (kuhn·DI·shuh·nuhr): a product that helps hair look smooth and shiny.

conflict: a disagreement.

consumer: a person who checks out health information; buys health products; uses health services; decides how to spend time and money; and chooses entertainment.

cool-down: five to ten minutes of easy exercise after a workout.

cooperate (koh·AH·puh·rayt): to work well with others toward a goal.

coordination (koh·awr·duh·NAY·shuhn): the ability to use more than one body part at a time.

cough medicine: helps stop a cough.

coward: a person who is not strong inside.

crown: the part of the tooth that sticks out above the gums.

cure: to make well.

cut: a break in the skin.

cuticle (KYOO·ti·kuhl): the skin around the nails.

D

dander: dead skin flakes.

decibel (DE·suh·buhl): a measure of the loudness of sounds.

decision (di·SI·zhuhn): a choice.

decongestant (DEE·kuhn·JES·tuhnt): helps clear a stuffy nose.

dental floss: a thin thread used to clean teeth.

deodorant: a product used under the arms to control body odor.

depressant (di·PRE·suhnt): a drug that slows down body functions.

Dietary Guidelines: suggested goals for eating to help you stay healthy and live longer.

dietitian (DY·uh·TI·shuhn): a person who plans healthful meals and runs a kitchen.

digestion (dy·JES·chuhn): a process of changing food you eat so it can be used by your body.

digestive (dy·JES·tiv) **system:** made up of organs that help your body use food.

disability (DI·suh·BI·luh·tee): something that changes a person's ability to do certain things.

disease: an illness that keeps your body from working as it should.

divorce: a legal way to end a marriage.

doctor: a person who is trained to treat people who are ill or injured.

doormat: a person whom other people walk all over.

drug: a substance that changes how your mind or body works.

drug abuse: the unsafe use of a medicine on purpose.

drug addiction: being unable to stop using a drug.

drug misuse: the unsafe use of a medicine that is not done on purpose.

dust mites: tiny insects that live in carpets, mattresses, and dust.

E

ear plugs: plugs put in the ears to block sounds.

ear protectors: coverings worn over the ears to block sounds.

emergency: a situation in which help is needed quickly.

emergency medical technician (TEK·ni·shuhn) **(EMT):** a person who takes care of people on the way to the hospital.

enamel: a hard white substance that covers the crown.

encyclopedia (in·SY·kluh·PEE·dee·uh): a set of books that has information on many subjects.

energy: the ability to do work.

entertainment (EN·tuhr·TAYN·muhnt): something that interests or amuses you.

environment (in·VY·ruhn·muhnt): everything that is around you.

F

family: a group of people who are related.

family and social health: how well you get along with your family and others.

family value: the importance of something to your family.

fast food restaurant: a place that serves food quickly.

fats: nutrients that are used for energy and to keep the body warm.

feelings: the ways you feel inside.

femurs (FEE·muhrz): your thigh bones.

fiber: the part of grains and plant foods that cannot be digested.

fight: a struggle between two or more people.

fire escape plan: a plan to get out safely if a fire breaks out.

firefighter: a person who puts out fires and helps people in emergencies.

first aid: the quick care given to a person who has been injured or suddenly becomes ill.

first aid kit: supplies needed to give first aid.

fitness skills: actions that help you do physical activities.

flexibility (flek·suh·BI·luh·tee): the ability to bend and move easily.

flood: the overflow of water onto dry land.

flossing: a way to remove food and plaque near the gums.

Food Guide Pyramid: a guide that tells how many servings are needed from each food group each day.

food label: a part of a package that lists the ingredients and nutrition information of a food.

friend who has special needs: a friend who has needs that are different from others.

friendly environment: an environment in which people get along, cooperate, and share space.

G

gang: a group of people who do violent things.

garbage: food and other things that are thrown out.

good character (KEHR·ik·tuhr): telling the truth, showing respect, and being fair.

gossip: saying unkind things about a person.

graffiti (grah·FEE·tee): writing on property.

grooming: taking care of your body and appearance.

Guidelines for Making Responsible Decisions™: six questions to ask to help you make a responsible decision.

gums: the pink tissue around a tooth.

H

harmful stress: stress that harms health or causes you to perform poorly.

head lice: tiny insects that lay eggs in the hair.

health: the condition of your body, mind, and relationships.

health behavior contract: a written plan to help you practice a life skill.

health helper: a person who helps you stay healthy.

health information: facts about health.

healthful entertainment: entertainment that promotes health.

healthful stress: stress that helps you perform well and stay healthy.

hearing aid: a small device that makes sounds louder.

hearing loss: being unable to hear some sounds.

heart: a muscular organ that pumps blood.

heart attack: a sudden lack of oxygen to the heart.

heart disease: a disease of the heart and blood vessels.

heart fitness: the condition of your heart and blood vessels.

helper T cell: a special kind of white blood cell.

heredity: the traits you get from your birth parents.

hero: a person you look up to because of something the person has done or does.

HIV: the germ that causes AIDS.

hobby: something you like to do in your spare time.

honest talk: saying exactly how you feel.

I

idea: a thought or belief.

illegal drugs: drugs that are against the law.

I-message: a healthful way to say or write about feelings.

infestation: having mites, ticks, lice, or worms.

inhalant (in·HAY·luhnt): a chemical that is breathed.

inhaler (in·HAY·luhr): a device that sprays medicine into a person's air passages.

injury: damage or harm done to a person.

J-K-L

joint: is the place where bones meet.

landfill: a place where waste is dumped and buried.

large intestine: the body organ through which solid waste passes.

learning disability: something that causes a person to have trouble learning.

life skill: a healthful action you learn and practice for life.

litter: trash that is thrown on land or in water.

loving actions: actions that show your special feelings for someone.

loving feelings: feelings you have toward someone you care about.

lungs: two organs that put oxygen into the blood and take carbon dioxide out of the blood.

M

marijuana (mehr·uh·WAH·nuh): a drug that harms memory and concentration.

medical assistant: a person who helps run a doctor's office.

medical record technician (TEK·ni·shuhn): a person who makes sure your health records are clear.

medicine: a drug used to treat an illness or injury.

memory: something from the past that you remember.

mental and emotional health: how well your mind works and how you show your feelings.

message: words or body movements used to say something to another person.

minerals: nutrients that are used to help your body work as it should.

mood: the way you feel at a certain time.

mouthguard: an object worn to protect the teeth and gums.

MSG: a substance used to flavor foods.

muscle (MUH·suhl): a tissue that allows your body to move.

muscle endurance (ihn·DOOR·unts): the ability to use your muscles for a long time.

muscle strength: the ability of your muscles to lift, pull, and push.

muscular (MUHS·kyuh·luhr) **system:** made up of all the muscles in your body.

N

nail polish: a coating to shine or color nails.

natural sugar: the sugar that is in foods and has not been added.

neighborhood: the small area in which you live.

nerves: groups of special cells in your body that carry messages from your sense organs to your brain.

nervous (NUHR·vuhs) **system:** made up of organs that control all your body actions.

newsgroup: a place on a computer system where people can write questions and read answers.

nicotine (NI·kuh·teen): a drug in tobacco that speeds up the body.

noise: sounds that make you feel uncomfortable or annoyed.

nose: an organ that draws air into your body and allows you to smell things.

nurse: a person who is trained to take care of sick or injured people and who is supervised by a doctor.

nutrient (NOO·tree·uhnt): a material in food that is used by the body.

O

organ: a body part made of different kinds of tissues.

organized (OR·guh·NYZD): to keep track of your time and your belongings.

over-the-counter (OTC) medicine: a medicine that you can buy without a doctor's order.

oxygen (AHK·si·juhn): a gas needed for you to live.

P-Q

pay back: to make good for loss or damage.

pay forward: to pay back for wrongdoing by doing something kind for someone else.

peer: someone who is your age.

permanent (PUHR·muh·nuhnt) **teeth:** a second set of teeth.

personal flotation device (PUHR·suhn·uhl floh·TAY·shuhn di·VYS): a device that helps you stay afloat.

personality: the blend of ways you look, think, act, and feel.

perspiration (PUHR·spuh·RAY·shuhn): a liquid made in sweat glands.

pharmacist (FAR·muh·sist): a person who gives out medicine your doctor prescribes.

pharmacy (FAR·muh·see): a place where prescription drugs are given out or sold.

physical fitness: having your body in top condition.

physical fitness plan: a written plan of physical activities you will do.

physical health: how well your body works.

plaque (PLAK): a sticky material that forms on teeth.

poison: a material that can harm you.

police officer: a person who keeps you safe by making sure people follow laws.

pollen: a powdery substance in plants that can get in the air.

pollution (puh·LOO·shuhn): substances in the environment that can harm health.

posture (PAHS·chuhr): the way you hold your body as you sit, stand, and move.

poultry: meat from chickens, turkeys, or other birds.

power: the ability to use strong muscles.

precycle: to keep from making trash.

prescription (pri·SKRIP·shuhn) **medicine:** a medicine that you can buy only if a doctor writes an order.

primary (PRY·MEHR·ee) **teeth:** first teeth.

proteins (PROH·teenz): nutrients that are used to grow and repair body cells.

puberty (PYOO·ber·tee): the stage in life when a person's body changes to become an adult.

pulp: the soft inner part of a tooth.

R

reaction time: the amount of time it takes your muscles to respond to a message from your brain.

recycle: to change trash so it can be used again.

reliable (ri·LY·uh·buhl) **information:** information that is based on scientific study.

remarry: to get married again.

resistance skills: ways to say NO to wrong decisions.

resources (REE·sohr·sez): things that occur in nature and are used to make other things.

respect: thinking highly of someone.

respiratory (RES·puh·ruh·TOR·ee) **system:** made up of organs that help you use the air you breathe.

responsible (ri·SPAHN·suh·buhl): to be in charge of doing something.

responsible decision: a choice you will be proud of.

ribs: the bones that cover and protect your heart and lungs.

root: the part of the tooth that holds it to the jawbone.

rule: a guide to help you do the right thing.

S

safety belt: the lap belt and the shoulder belt.

safety equipment: equipment that helps keep you from getting hurt during sports.

safety seal: an unbroken seal to show a container has not been opened.

saliva (suh·LY·vuh): a liquid in your mouth that softens food.

salivary (SA·luh·VEHR·ee) **glands:** organs that make saliva.

scabies: a skin infestation caused by a mite.

school nurse: takes care of students who get sick or hurt at school.

scrape: the tearing or wearing away of skin.

secondhand smoke: the smoke from other people's cigarettes and cigars.

self-concept: the feeling you have about yourself.

self-control: being able to hold back from doing something you should not do.

self-esteem: the way you feel about yourself.

self-respect: thinking highly of yourself.

set limits: to be clear as to what is OK and what is not OK with you.

shampoo: a soap that cleans the hair.

side effect: an unwanted feeling or illness after taking a medicine.

sign language: a way to communicate by using the hands and arms instead of speaking.

silverware: knives, forks, and spoons.

skeletal (SKE·luh·tuhl) **system:** the group of bones in your body.

skill: something you do that takes practice.

skin: the organ that covers your body.

skull: the bones on your head and the bones of your face.

small intestine: an organ that breaks down most of the food you eat into substances your body cells can use.

smokeless tobacco: tobacco that is not burned.

snack: food eaten between meals.

speed: the ability to move fast.

spinal cord: a long column of nerve cells that attaches to your brain.

starches: carbohydrates that provide energy that lasts a long time.

stimulant (STIM·yuh·luhnt): a drug that speeds up body functions.

stomach: an organ that releases special juices to break down food.

stranger (STRAYN·juhr): someone you do not know well.

strep throat: a sore throat caused by a kind of bacteria.

stress: the response to any demand on your mind and body.

stressor (STRE·suhr): anything that causes stress.

stroke: a condition that is caused by a blocked or broken blood vessel in the brain.

study: to review and practice the things you have learned.

sugars: carbohydrates that provide quick energy.

sunburn: a burn on the skin caused by too much sun.

symptom: a change from normal in a person's health.

T

table manners: polite ways to eat.

tar: a brown, sticky substance in tobacco that is harmful.

television addiction: being unable to stop watching TV when you should be doing something else.

thrift shop: a shop that sells used items.

throat: the passage between your mouth and your windpipe.

tissue (TI·shoo): a group of cells that work together to do a special job.

tobacco (tuh·BA·koh): a plant that contains chemicals that are harmful to health.

tornado: a high speed windstorm that is shaped like a funnel.

true friend: a friend whose actions are responsible and caring.

U

unloving actions: actions that harm other people.

unsafe touch: a touch that is not right.

V

vaccine (vak·SEEN): a substance made with dead or weak germs.

veins: blood vessels that bring blood back to your heart.

vertebrae (VUHR·tuh·bray): 26 bones that make up your spine, or backbone.

veterinarian (VE·tuh·ruh·NEHR·ee·uhn): a doctor who takes care of animals.

violence: harm done to yourself, others or property.

viruses (VY·ruh·suhz): germs that are much smaller than bacteria.

visual environment: everything you see often.

vitamins (VY·tuh·muhnz): nutrients that help your body use proteins, carbohydrates, and fats.

volunteer: someone who works without pay.

W-X-Y-Z

warm-up: three to five minutes of easy physical activity before a workout.

waste-treatment plant: a place where water is cleaned.

water: a nutrient that is used for body processes.

water pollution: substances in water that make it unclean and harmful.

water-treatment plant: a place where water is treated and made safe to drink.

weapon: an object used to harm someone.

Web site: information put on the Web by a certain group.

willpower: the strength you need to do the right thing.

windpipe: a tube that goes from your throat to your lungs.

World Wide Web (Web): a computer system that lets a person find information, pictures, and text.